Comparative Effectiveness Review

Number 108

Migraine in Children: Preventive Pharmacologic Treatments

Prepared for:
Agency for Healthcare Research and Quality
U.S. Department of Health and Human Services
540 Gaither Road
Rockville, MD 20850
www.ahrq.gov

Contract No. 290-07-10064-I

Prepared by:
Minnesota Evidence-based Practice Center
Minneapolis, MN

Investigators:
Tatyana A. Shamliyan, M.D., M.S.
Robert L. Kane, M.D.
Rema Ramakrishnan, M.P.H.
Frederick R. Taylor, M.D.

AHRQ Publication No. 13-EHC065-EF
June 2013

This report is based on research conducted by the Minnesota Evidence-based Practice Center (EPC) under contract to the Agency for Healthcare Research and Quality (AHRQ), Rockville, MD (Contract No. 290-07-10064-I). The findings and conclusions in this document are those of the authors, who are responsible for its contents; the findings and conclusions do not necessarily represent the views of AHRQ. Therefore, no statement in this report should be construed as an official position of AHRQ or of the U.S. Department of Health and Human Services.

The information in this report is intended to help health care decisionmakers—patients and clinicians, health system leaders, and policymakers, among others—make well-informed decisions and thereby improve the quality of health care services. This report is not intended to be a substitute for the application of clinical judgment. Anyone who makes decisions concerning the provision of clinical care should consider this report in the same way as any medical reference and in conjunction with all other pertinent information, i.e., in the context of available resources and circumstances presented by individual patients.

This report may be used, in whole or in part, as the basis for development of clinical practice guidelines and other quality enhancement tools, or as a basis for reimbursement and coverage policies. AHRQ or U.S. Department of Health and Human Services endorsement of such derivative products may not be stated or implied.

This document is in the public domain and may be used and reprinted without special permission. Citation of the source is appreciated.

Persons using assistive technology may not be able to fully access information in this report. For assistance contact EffectiveHealthCare@ahrq.hhs.gov.

Suggested citation: Shamliyan TA, Kane RL, Ramakrishnan R, Taylor FR. Migraine in Children: Preventive Pharmacologic Treatments. Comparative Effectiveness Review No. 108. (Prepared by the University of Minnesota Evidence-based Practice Center under Contract No. 290-2007-10064-I.) AHRQ Publication No. 13-EHC065-EF. Rockville, MD: Agency for Healthcare Research and Quality; June 2013. www.effectivehealthcare.ahrq.gov/reports/final.cfm.

Preface

The Agency for Healthcare Research and Quality (AHRQ), through its Evidence-based Practice Centers (EPCs), sponsors the development of systematic reviews to assist public- and private-sector organizations in their efforts to improve the quality of health care in the United States. These reviews provide comprehensive, science-based information on common, costly medical conditions, and new health care technologies and strategies.

Systematic reviews are the building blocks underlying evidence-based practice; they focus attention on the strength and limits of evidence from research studies about the effectiveness and safety of a clinical intervention. In the context of developing recommendations for practice, systematic reviews can help clarify whether assertions about the value of the intervention are based on strong evidence from clinical studies. For more information about AHRQ EPC systematic reviews, see www.effectivehealthcare.ahrq.gov/reference/purpose.cfm.

AHRQ expects that these systematic reviews will be helpful to health plans, providers, purchasers, government programs, and the health care system as a whole. Transparency and stakeholder input are essential to the Effective Health Care Program. Please visit the Web site (www.effectivehealthcare.ahrq.gov) to see draft research questions and reports or to join an email list to learn about new program products and opportunities for input.

We welcome comments on this systematic review. They may be sent by mail to the Task Order Officer named below at: Agency for Healthcare Research and Quality, 540 Gaither Road, Rockville, MD 20850, or by email to epc@ahrq.hhs.gov.

Carolyn M. Clancy, M.D.
Director
Agency for Healthcare Research and Quality

Jean Slutsky, P.A., M.S.P.H.
Director, Center for Outcomes and Evidence
Agency for Healthcare Research and Quality

Stephanie Chang, M.D., M.P.H.
Director, EPC Program
Center for Outcomes and Evidence
Agency for Healthcare Research and Quality

Suchitra Iyer, Ph.D.
Task Order Officer
Center for Outcomes and Evidence
Agency for Healthcare Research and Quality

Acknowledgments

The authors gratefully acknowledge the following individuals for their contributions to this project. We would like to thank the librarians, Judy Stanke, M.A., and Delbert Reed, Ph.D., for their contributions to the literature search; Jae-Young Choi, M.H.P.A., Ph.D., Jennifer Biggs Miller, P.T., M.P.H., C.W.S., and Shi-Yi Wang, M.D., M.S., Ph.D., for their assistance with the literature search and data abstraction; Jeannine Ouellette for her help in writing the report; Marilyn Eells for editing and formatting the report; and Christa Prodzinski, R.N., and Kirsten Johnson, B.S., for assistance with data entry, quality control, and formatting tables. We would like to thank Thomas Trikalinos, M.D., Ph.D., and Gerta Rücker, Ph.D., for their statistical advice in arcsine transformation of the data.

Key Informants

In designing the study questions, the EPC consulted several Key Informants who represent the end-users of research. The EPC sought the Key Informant input on the priority areas for research and synthesis. Key Informants are not involved in the analysis of the evidence or the writing of the report. Therefore, in the end, study questions, design, methodological approaches, and/or conclusions do not necessarily represent the views of individual Key Informants.

Key Informants must disclose any financial conflicts of interest greater than $10,000 and any other relevant business or professional conflicts of interest. Because of their role as end-users, individuals with potential conflicts may be retained. The TOO and the EPC work to balance, manage, or mitigate any conflicts of interest.

The list of Key Informants who participated in developing this report follows:

Thomas Becker, M.D., M.B.A.
Medica Health Plans
Minnetonka, MN

Roger K. Cady, M.D.
Headache Care Center
Springfield, MO

Robert Dalton
National Headache Foundation
Chicago, IL

Lida Etermad, Pharm.D., M.S.
United Healthcare
Edina, MN

Andrew D. Hershey, M.D., Ph.D.
University of Cincinnati College of Medicine
Cincinnati, OH

Brady Patrick-Lake, M.F.S.
Consumer representative
Erie, CO

Alan M. Rapoport, M.D.
David Geffen School of Medicine, UCLA
Los Angeles, CA

Stephen D. Silberstein, M.D., FACP
Jefferson Headache Center
Philadelphia, PA

Technical Expert Panel

In designing the study questions and methodology at the outset of this report, the EPC consulted several technical and content experts. Broad expertise and perspectives were sought. Divergent and conflicted opinions are common and perceived as healthy scientific discourse that results in a thoughtful, relevant systematic review. Therefore, in the end, study questions, design, methodologic approaches, and/or conclusions do not necessarily represent the views of individual technical and content experts.

Technical Experts must disclose any financial conflicts of interest greater than $10,000 and any other relevant business or professional conflicts of interest. Because of their unique clinical or content expertise, individuals with potential conflicts may be retained. The TOO and the EPC work to balance, manage, or mitigate any potential conflicts of interest identified.

The list of Technical Experts who participated in developing this report follows:

Andrew Blumenfeld, M.D.
Kaiser Permanente
San Diego, CA

Alan M. Rapoport, M.D.
David Geffen School of Medicine, UCLA
Los Angeles, CA

Roger K. Cady, M.D.
Headache Care Center
Springfield, MO

Stephen D. Silberstein, M.D., FACP
Jefferson Headache Center
Philadelphia, PA

Andrew D. Hershey, M.D., Ph.D.
University of Cincinnati College of Medicine
Cincinnati, OH

Peer Reviewers

Prior to publication of the final evidence report, EPCs sought input from independent Peer Reviewers without financial conflicts of interest. However, the conclusions and synthesis of the scientific literature presented in this report does not necessarily represent the views of individual reviewers.

Peer Reviewers must disclose any financial conflicts of interest greater than $10,000 and any other relevant business or professional conflicts of interest. Because of their unique clinical or content expertise, individuals with potential nonfinancial conflicts may be retained. The TOO and the EPC work to balance, manage, or mitigate any potential nonfinancial conflicts of interest identified.

The list of Peer Reviewers follows:

Andrew Blumenfeld, M.D.
Kaiser Permanente
San Diego, CA

Rochelle Fu, Ph.D.
Oregon Evidence-based Practice Center
Portland, OR

Frederick Freitag, D.O., FAHS
Baylor Research Institute
Dallas, TX

Brady Patrick-Lake, M.F.S.
Consumer representative
Erie, CO

Migraine in Children: Preventive Pharmacologic Treatments

Structured Abstract

Objectives. To assess the comparative effectiveness and safety of preventive pharmacologic treatments for community-dwelling children with episodic or chronic migraine.

Data sources. We searched major electronic bibliographic databases, including Medline® and Cochrane Central Register of Controlled Trials, and trial registries up to May 20, 2012.

Review methods. We performed a systematic review of original studies published in English that examined episodic or chronic migraine and rates of complete cessation or reduction of monthly migraine frequency by ≥50 percent, reduction in migraine-related disability, and improvement in quality of life with off-label drugs. (No preventive drugs were approved in children.) Also eligible were studies that compared drugs with nonpharmacologic interventions or drug management programs. We calculated absolute risk differences, pooled them with random-effects models, and calculated numbers of outcome events attributable to treatment effects per 1,000 treated.

Results. Prevention of episodic migraine in children was examined in 24 publications of randomized controlled trials (RCTs) that enrolled 1,578 children and in 16 nonrandomized studies. Evidence was low strength due to risk of bias and imprecision. Propranolol was estimated to result in complete cessation of migraine attacks in 713 per 1,000 children treated (95-percent confidence interval [CI], 452 to 974) (one RCT). Trazodone (one RCT) and nimodipine (one RCT) decreased migraine days more effectively than placebo. Topiramate (two RCTs), divalproex (one RCT), and clonidine (one RCT) were no more effective than placebo in preventing migraine. Sodium valproate demonstrated no significant differences for migraine prevention or migraine-related disability compared with propranolol (two RCTs) or topiramate (one RCT). Metoprolol tended to be less effective than stress management in preventing migraine or reducing migraine severity (one RCT). Propranolol had less effect than self-hypnosis on absolute number of migraine attacks (one RCT). Multidisciplinary drug management was more effective than usual care in preventing migraine in children and adolescents (one RCT), but the effect was not sustained at 6 months. Divalproex sodium (one RCT) resulted in treatment discontinuation due to adverse effects more often than placebo. Treatment discontinuation due to adverse effects did not differ between topiramate (two RCTs), trazodone (one RCT), propranolol (one RCT), or clonidine (one RCT) and placebo. Topiramate increased risk of paresthesia, upper respiratory tract infection, and weight loss. No RCTs examined prevention of chronic migraine in children.

Conclusions. Limited low-strength evidence suggests that propranolol was more effective than placebo for preventing episodic migraine in children, with no bothersome adverse effects that could lead to treatment discontinuation. Long-term preventive benefits are unknown both for drugs and nonpharmacologic interventions. No studies examined quality of life or provided evidence for individualized treatment decisions. Future randomized trials of drugs with favorable benefits-to-harms ratio in adults are needed to identify effective and safe treatments to prevent episodic and chronic migraine in children.

Contents

Figures

Appendixes

Appendix A. Literature Search
Appendix B. Ongoing Studies of Migraine Prevention in Children
Appendix C. Analytical Framework
Appendix D. Evidence Tables
Appendix E. Excluded Studies

Executive Summary

Introduction

The Agency for Healthcare Research and Quality (AHRQ) commissioned the Minnesota Evidence-based Practice Center (EPC) to conduct a review of preventive pharmacologic treatments for migraine. This review of migraine prevention is presented in two parallel reports, one focusing on children and one on adults. Here we address migraine prevention in children 6 to 18 years old.

According to the International Classification of Headache Disorders, second edition (ICHD-II), migraine is a common disabling primary headache disorder manifesting in attacks that last from 4 to 72 hours.[1,2] Migraine headaches range from moderate to very severe[3] and are sometimes debilitating.[4] In the United States, episodic migraine affects 5 percent of boys[5,6] and 7.7 percent of girls.[7,8] According to the American Migraine Prevalence and Prevention Study (a large national cohort study), childhood migraine is more prevalent in lower income families, and adolescent migraine is more prevalent in whites than in African Americans.[7]

Migraine frequency is classified as either episodic or chronic[2] according to the number of monthly migraine days, with episodic being <15 days, and chronic being ≥15 days. Migraine may also be described as chronic when attacks recur over long periods of time. Chronic migraine affects 2 percent of children and adolescents.[9]

Both migraine types significantly affect children's physical, psychological, and social well-being, and can impose serious lifestyle restrictions.[9] The majority of adolescents with chronic migraine have some related disability.[9] Yet, according to the Chronic Daily Headache in Adolescents Study (C-dAS), less than half of adolescents with chronic migraine had visited a health care provider for the condition, and fewer than one in five had taken medications to prevent headaches during the previous month.[9] Approximately 31 percent of children with migraine had missed at least 1 day of school in the previous 3 months due to migraine.[10] Childhood migraine has also been shown to impair learning and school productivity by 50 percent or more.[10]

Migraine treatments aim either to ameliorate acute attacks or prevent attacks. Many children with frequent or severe migraine need preventive treatment. Our review focuses on preventive treatments for childhood migraine. The Food and Drug Administration (FDA) has approved no drugs for migraine prevention in children; therefore, pediatricians prescribe drugs approved for adults or off-label drugs (approved for clinical conditions other than migraine prevention). The off-label drug classes that were used cause common and serious adverse effects, including metabolic and hormonal abnormalities.[11-15] Preventive pharmacologic treatments for migraine in children should be based on the efficacy and safety of the drugs, whether approved for adults or used off label.

Preventive treatment aims to eliminate headache pain. Often, however, some pain persists; therefore, treatment success is usually defined by a decrease in migraine frequency of ≥50 percent after 3 months.[3] In addition to pain relief, preventive drugs can decrease severity of migraine attacks and reduce restrictions in daily activities and schooling.

Scope

Our review focuses on the comparative effectiveness and safety of drugs (approved for use in the United States) for preventing migraine attacks in children seen in ambulatory care settings. Our results may help inform treatment recommendations.

During the topic refinement stage, we solicited input from Key Informants representing medical professional societies/clinicians in the areas of neurology and primary care, consumers, scientific experts, and payers to help define the Key Questions.[16] The Key Questions were then posted for public comment for 4 weeks from April 12, 2012, to May 10, 2012, and the comments received were considered in the development of the research protocol. We next convened a Technical Expert Panel (TEP) comprising clinical, content, and methodological experts to provide input in defining populations, interventions, comparisons, and outcomes, and in identifying particular studies or databases to search. The Key Informants and members of the TEP were required to disclose any financial conflicts of interest greater than $10,000 and any other relevant business or professional conflicts. Any potential conflicts of interest were balanced or mitigated. Neither Key Informants nor members of the TEP performed analysis of any kind, nor did any of them contribute to the writing of this report. Members of the TEP were invited to provide feedback on an initial draft of the review protocol, which was then refined based on their input and that of outside reviewers, reviewed by AHRQ, and posted for public access on the AHRQ Effective Health Care Web site.

We chose not to synthesize studies of the drug flunarizine because the FDA has not approved it. Efficacy of nonpharmacologic preventive treatments was beyond our scope. We conducted a comprehensive literature review following the principles in the "Methods Guide for Effectiveness and Comparative Effectiveness Reviews" (Methods Guide) developed by the AHRQ EPC Program[17,18] and the Preferred Reporting Items for Systematic Reviews and Meta-Analyses (PRISMA) guidelines for systematic reviews. We registered the protocol for our review (protocol registration number CRD42011001858, available at www.crd.york.ac.uk/prospero/display_record.asp?ID=CRD42011001858).[19]

Key Questions

Key Question 1: What are the efficacy and comparative effectiveness of pharmacologic treatments for preventing migraine attacks in children?

  a. How do preventive pharmacologic treatments affect patient-centered and intermediate outcomes when compared with placebo or no active treatment?
  b. How do preventive pharmacologic treatments affect patient-centered and intermediate outcomes when compared with active pharmacologic treatments?
  c. How do preventive pharmacologic treatments affect patient-centered and intermediate outcomes when compared with active nonpharmacologic treatments?
  d. How do preventive pharmacologic treatments combined with nondrug treatments affect patient-centered and intermediate outcomes when compared with pharmacologic treatments alone?
  e. How might dosing regimens or duration of treatments influence the effects of the treatments on patient-centered outcomes? How might approaches to drug management (such as patient-care teams, integrated care, coordinated care, patient education, drug surveillance, or interactive drug monitoring) influence results?

Key Question 2: What are the comparative harms from pharmacologic treatments for preventing migraine attacks in children?

  a. What are the harms from preventive pharmacologic treatments when compared with placebo or no active treatment?
  b. What are the harms from preventive pharmacologic treatments when compared with active pharmacologic treatments?
  c. How might approaches to drug management (such as patient-care teams, integrated care, coordinated care, patient education, drug surveillance, or interactive drug monitoring) improve safety of the treatments?

Key Question 3: Which characteristics of children predict the effectiveness and safety of pharmacologic treatments for preventing migraine attacks?

Methods

We followed an a priori research protocol that we developed with the clinical and methodological input of the TEP. The protocol followed the Effective Health Care Program's Methods Guide.

Literature Search Strategy

We used the standard methods developed by the AHRQ EPC program.[17,18] We searched several bibliographic databases, including MEDLINE® (via Ovid and PubMed®), the Cochrane Library, SCIRUS, the FDA Web site, clinical trial registries, and reference lists of published reviews to find ongoing, completed, and published trials of migraine prevention in children.

Eligibility

Three investigators independently determined study eligibility, resolving disagreement in discussions until consensus was achieved.[20,21]

We determined eligibility according to the PICOTS (population, intervention, comparator, outcomes, timing, and settings) framework. We defined the target population as community-dwelling children with episodic migraine, chronic daily headache, or chronic migraine defined according to criteria set by the International Headache Society.[22] We formulated a list of eligible interventions after discussions with Key Informants and technical experts and after consideration of public comments. Eligible comparators included pharmacologic, nonpharmacologic, and combined preventive treatments. We defined eligible intermediate and patient-centered outcomes (presented in the analytical framework, Figure A).

To assess benefits, we included randomized controlled trials (RCTs) published in English up to May 20, 2012. We reviewed original clinical studies that included children with migraine, comorbid headache disorders, or tension headache as long as migraine prevention was examined. To assess harms of treatments we included published and unpublished RCTs and nonrandomized studies of the adverse effects of drugs in children with migraine.[20] We defined harms as the totality of all possible adverse consequences of an intervention. We analyzed harms regardless of how authors perceived the causality of treatments.

We excluded studies of treatments aimed at acute migraine attacks, studies that involved patients with migraine variants (e.g., basilar migraine, childhood periodic syndromes, retinal migraine, complicated migraine, and ophthalmoplegic migraine), and patients who were hospitalized or in emergency rooms. We also excluded hemiplegic migraine, a pathophysiologically distinct disorder with its own classification. We excluded studies that included some pediatric patients with migraine but did not separately report the outcomes, studies that involved surgical treatments for migraine, preclinical pharmacokinetic studies of eligible drugs, studies that examined the pathophysiology of migraine and reported instrumental measurements or biochemical outcomes, and studies that examined eligible drugs on populations with other diseases. Studies evaluating the efficacy of nonpharmacologic treatments or economic outcomes were beyond the scope of this review.

Data Extraction

Researchers used standardized forms to extract data (available at https://netfiles.umn.edu/xythoswfs/webui/_xy-21041343_1-t_zdhvSpvy). For each trial, one reviewer extracted the data and a second reviewer checked the abstracted data for accuracy. We assessed errors by comparing established ranges for each variable and data charts from the original articles. Any detected discrepancies were discussed.

We abstracted the information relevant to the PICOTS framework (Figure A). We abstracted minimum datasets to reproduce the results presented by the authors. For categorical variables we abstracted the number of events among treatment groups to calculate rates, relative risk, and absolute risk differences (ARDs). Means and standard deviations of continuous variables were abstracted to calculate mean differences with a 95% confidence interval (CI).

For RCTs in the quantitative analysis set, we abstracted the number randomized to each treatment group as the denominator to calculate estimates by applying intention-to-treat principles. We abstracted the time when the outcomes were assessed as weeks from randomization and time of followup after treatments.

We abstracted inclusion and exclusion criteria, drug regimen and doses, and patient characteristics that can modify treatment effects, including demographics, baseline frequency, severity, and prior treatment status. We abstracted the migraine definition used in each study. We abstracted sponsorship of the studies and conflict of interest of the authors.

Figure A. Analytical framework

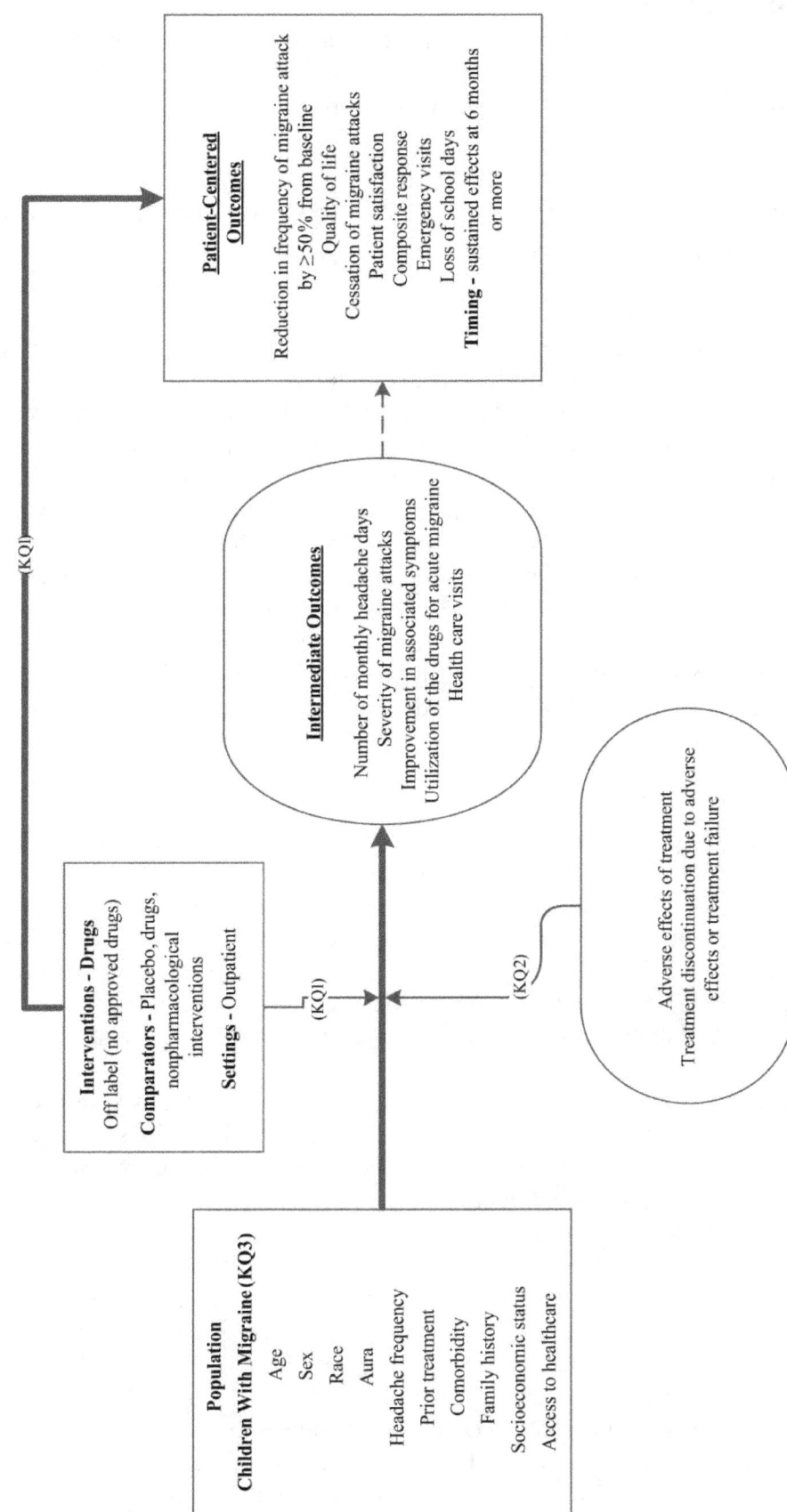

Key Question 1: What are the efficacy and comparative effectiveness of pharmacologic treatments for preventing migraine attacks in children?
Key Question 2: What are the comparative harms from pharmacologic treatments for preventing migraine attacks in children?
Key Question 3: Which characteristics of children predict the effectiveness and safety of pharmacologic treatments for preventing migraine attacks?

Risk-of-Bias Assessment

We evaluated the risk of bias in individual studies according to study design using criteria from the Cochrane risk-of-bias tool in interventional studies:

- Random allocation of the subjects to treatment groups
- Masking of the treatment status
- Adequacy of allocation concealment
- Adequacy of randomization according to baseline similarity of the subjects in treatment groups by demographics, migraine frequency and severity, and response to previous treatments
- Intention-to-treat principles
- Selective outcome reporting when compared with the posted protocols (when trials were registered) or with the methods sections in the articles

We assumed a low risk of bias when RCTs met all of the risk-of-bias criteria, a medium risk of bias if one criterion was not met, and a high risk of bias if two or more criteria were not met. We concluded an unknown risk of bias for studies with poorly reported risk-of-bias criteria. Since all outcomes in the review were self-reported, masking of outcome assessment was not essential in evaluating risk of bias, but masking of treatment was. Masking of treatment status was not feasible for RCTs that examined nondrug therapies as comparators; therefore, we did not include it in risk-of-bias assessment for those studies. We appraised risk of bias in nonrandomized studies according to selection, attrition, and detection biases.

We evaluated disclosure of conflict of interest by the authors of individual studies and funding sources but did not use this information to downgrade the quality of individual studies.

Data Synthesis

We summarized the results into evidence tables. We focused on the patient-centered outcomes of reduction in migraine attack rate by ≥ 50 percent from baseline, quality of life, patient satisfaction, and composite outcomes, which included migraine frequency and severity. We incorporated risk of bias in individual studies into the evidence synthesis using individual risk-of-bias criteria rather than a global score or a ranking category of overall risk of bias.

Using Meta-Analyst and STATA® software, we calculated the relative risk and absolute risk difference from the abstracted events and the mean differences in continuous variables from the reported means and standard deviations. We evaluated statistical significance at a 95% confidence level.

Pooling criteria for Key Questions 1 and 2 included the requirement that studies examined the same active drug treatments and comparators and used the same definitions of the outcomes. We calculated Cohen standardized mean differences for different continuous measures of the same outcome. We did not pool RCTs with nonrandomized studies or studies of different pharmacologic drug classes with each other.

We tested consistency in the results by comparing the direction and strength of the association. We assessed heterogeneity in results with chi-square and I-squared tests. Using the random-effects model, we incorporated into the pooled analysis any differences between trials in patient populations, baseline rates of the outcomes, dosage of drugs, and other factors.

We calculated the number needed to treat to achieve one event of a patient-centered outcome as the reciprocal of statistically significant ARDs in rates of outcome events in the active and control groups. We calculated means and 95% CIs for the number needed to treat as the reciprocal of pooled ARDs when ARDs were significant. The number of avoided or excess events per population of 1,000 was the difference between the two event rates multiplied by 1,000.

We focused on direct comparisons and synthesized evidence from head-to-head comparative effectiveness studies. We did not attempt to conduct network meta-analysis of sparse data.

Grading the Evidence for Each Key Question

We assessed strength of evidence according to risk of bias, consistency, directness, and precision for patient-centered outcomes, including 100 percent or ≥50 percent reduction in monthly migraine frequency, patient global assessment of treatment success, rates of clinically important improvement in migraine-related disability, and quality of life.[23] We also assessed treatment discontinuation due to harms. We defined treatment effect estimates as precise when pooled estimates had reasonably narrow 95% CIs or pooled samples had ≥300 events.[24] We did not include justification of the sample size into grading of the evidence, nor did we conduct post hoc statistical power analysis. We defined reporting bias as either publication bias, selective outcomes reporting, or multiple publication bias. We did not perform formal statistical tests to quantify the biases.

When evidence was available, we assessed dose-response association and strength of association in nonrandomized studies. We evaluated the strength of the association a priori, defining a large effect as having relative risk >2 and a very large effect as having relative risk >5.[21] We defined low magnitude of effect as having relative risk that was significant but <2.

We defined high strength of evidence on the basis of consistent findings from well-designed RCTs. We downgraded strength of evidence to moderate if one of the four criteria for strength of evidence (risk of bias, directness, consistency, and precision) was not met. We downgraded strength of evidence to low if two or more criteria were not met. We assigned a low level of evidence to nonrandomized studies and upgraded strength of evidence for strong or dose-response associations. We defined evidence as insufficient when a single study with high risk of bias examined treatment effects or associations.

Our presentation of results includes reproducible statistical estimates of treatment effects and strength-of-evidence evaluation of benefits and harms for informed decisionmaking.

Assessing Applicability

We estimated applicability of the sample by evaluating the selection of children with migraine.[25] Studies of community-dwelling children who received drug treatments with 6 months or more followup had high applicability, as did large observational cohorts based on national registries, population-based effectiveness trials, and nationally representative administrative and clinical databases.

Results

Of 510 retrieved references, we excluded 104 as not relevant at screening, and we reviewed full texts of 312. Of these, we included 24 references of RCTs, two abstracts of RCTs, and 16 nonrandomized studies. We did not grade the strength of evidence from two flunarizine RCTs because the FDA has not approved this drug (although it is commonly used outside the United States).

Of 14 completed clinical trials registered in ClinicalTrials.gov, 4 were published. Publications occurred 1.8±1.2 years after study completion. Completion dates were missing for three completed unpublished studies of divalproex. Of nine phase 3 studies involving exclusively children, none posted the results on ClinicalTrials.gov. The results were not available for 4,001 subjects enrolled in studies involving children or 1,093 children enrolled in exclusively pediatric studies.

Eligible trials enrolled on average 76 children (14 to 305) and aimed to examine prevention of episodic migraine and adverse effects. Few trials reported statistical power to detect statistically significant differences in outcomes.

Applicability

The results from the eligible studies were applicable to the target population. Most trials were conducted in Western countries and recruited children and adolescents in clinics. Only two trials recruited participants from the community. White girls made up more than half of all enrolled subjects. Many enrolled subjects were overweight according to their mean age and mean body mass index. Enrolled subjects had migraines for an average 3.6 years and suffered from an average of eight monthly migraine attacks. Most trials defined migraine according to the International Headache Society diagnostic criteria. Reporting of other characteristics of children was poor. More than half the trials did not report family history of migraine, children's socioeconomic status, baseline comorbidity, prior treatments, overuse of drugs for acute migraine, or adherence to assigned treatments. The trials lasted an average of 20 weeks (ranging from 6 to 35 weeks). Attrition rates with drugs averaged 6.9 percent.

Risk of Bias

Of all included trials, we concluded low risk of bias in nine RCTs, medium risk of bias in six RCTs, and unclear risk of bias in five RCTs. Most trials were double blind; however, randomization was adequate in just 12 trials. Risk of bias was associated with the journals of publication and with funding of the trials. Industry-funded RCTs had lower risk of bias than trials funded by grants or by combined or other sources.

We concluded high risk of bias in 16 nonrandomized studies that failed to address selection bias in their analyses.

Key Question 1. What are the efficacy and comparative effectiveness of pharmacologic treatments for preventing migraine attacks in children?

Key Question 1a. How do preventive pharmacologic treatments affect patient-centered and intermediate outcomes when compared with placebo or no active treatment?

Tables A and B present: (1) information from included RCTs on reduction in migraine frequency by ≥50 percent and treatment discontinuation due to adverse effects, (2) strength of evidence, and (3) number of events attributable to drug administration per 1,000 treated children. Table C presents our conclusions about effectiveness of pharmacologic treatments for preventing episodic migraine in children. Eligible trials defined clinically important migraine prevention as a complete cessation of migraine attacks and a reduction in monthly migraine frequency by either ≥50 or 75 percent. Here we present the effects of the drugs on patient-centered and intermediate outcomes.

Table A. Effects of preventive pharmacologic treatments on reduction in monthly migraine attacks

Outcome	Active	Control	RCTs	Children	Rate Active, %	Rate Control, %	Relative Risk (95% CI)	Absolute Risk Difference (95% CI)	Number Needed To Treat (95% CI)	Attributable Events per 1,000 Treated (95% CI)	Strength of Evidence (Reason for Lowering)
Complete cessation of headache attacks	**Propranolol**	**Placebo**	**1**	**28**	**84.6**	**13.0**	**6.3 (1.7 to 23.5)**	**0.71 (0.45 to 0.97)**	**1 (1 to 2)**	**713 (452 to 974)**	**Low** (imprecision in relative risk)
	Clonidine	Placebo	1	57	10.7	24.1	0.4 (0.1 to 1.5)	-0.13 (-0.33 to 0.06)	NS	NS	Low (imprecision)
	Sodium valproate	Propranolol	2	183	17.1	15.4	1.2 (0.6 to 2.2)	0.02 (-0.09 to 0.12)	NS	NS	Low (medium risk of bias, imprecision)
Reduction by ≥50% in migraine attack frequency	Topiramate	Placebo	2	298	58.2	45.7	1.3 (0.9 to 1.8)	0.15 (-0.06 to 0.37)	NS	NS	Moderate (medium risk of bias)
Reduction by ≥50% in migraine attack frequency	Divalproex sodium	Placebo	1	305	49.0	45.0	1.1 (0.8 to 1.5)	0.04 (-0.12 to 0.20)	NS	NS	Low (imprecision)
Reduction by ≥75% in migraine attack frequency	Propranolol	Placebo	1	28	7.7	0.0	3.4 (0.2 to 77.6)	0.08 (-0.11 to 0.26)	NS	NS	Low (imprecision)
1–2 migraine frequency/month	Clonidine	Placebo	1	57	32.1	27.6	1.2 (0.5 to 2.6)	0.05 (-0.19 to 0.28)	NS	NS	Low (imprecision)
Reduction by ≥50% in migraine attack frequency	Sodium valproate	Propranolol	2	183	69.5	74.3	0.9 (0.7 to 1.2)	-0.07 (-0.30 to 0.15)	NS	NS	Low (medium risk of bias, imprecision)

Table A. Effects of preventive pharmacologic treatments on reduction in monthly migraine attacks (continued)

Outcome	Active	Control	RCTs	Children	Rate Active, %	Rate Control, %	Relative Risk (95% CI)	Absolute Risk Difference (95% CI)	Number Needed To Treat (95% CI)	Attributable Events per 1,000 Treated (95% CI)	Strength of Evidence (Reason for Lowering)
Reduction by ≥50% in the headache index[a]	**Metoprolol**[b]	**Progressive relaxation training + stress management**	**1**	**28**	**38.5**	**80.0**	0.5 (0.2 to 1.0)	**-0.42 (-0.75 to -0.08)**	**-2 (-12 to -1)**	**-415 (-748 to -82)**	**Low** (unclear risk of bias, imprecision)
	Metoprolol	Cephalic vasomotor feedback + stress management	1	28	38.5	53.3	0.7 (0.3 to 1.7)	-0.15 (-0.51 to 0.22)	NS	NS	Low (unclear risk of bias, imprecision)
Reduction in need for temporary drug therapy for single attacks	Clonidine	Placebo	1	57	50.0	34.5	1.5 (0.8 to 2.7)	0.16 (-0.10 to 0.41)	NS	NS	Low (imprecision)
Improvement in Pediatric Migraine Disability Assessment Score	Topiramate	Sodium valproate	1	48	NA	NA	Mean difference -0.9 (-5.6 to 3.8)		NS	NS	Low (unclear risk of bias, imprecision)

CI = confidence interval; NA = not applicable; NS = not significant (number needed to treat and number of attributable events were calculated for statistically significant differences); RCT = randomized controlled trial

[a]Intensity of headache episodes.

[b]Bold = significant differences at 95% CI when the 95% CI of attributable events does not include 0.

Table B. Treatment discontinuation due to adverse effects with migraine preventive drugs versus placebo in children

Drug	RCTs	Children	Rate With Drug, %	Rate With Placebo, %	Relative Risk (95% CI)	Absolute Risk Difference (95% CI)	Number Needed To Treat (95% CI)	Attributable Events per 1,000 Treated (95% CI)	Strength of Evidence (Reason for Lowering)
Divalproex sodium, 1,000 mg[a]	**1**	**148**	**9.3**	**1.4**	**6.8 (0.9 to 54)**	**0.08 (0.01 to 0.16)**	**13 (7 to 111)**	**80 (9 to 151)**	**Low** (imprecision)
Topiramate, 50-200 mg	2	298	7	3.5	2.1 (0.7 to 6.3)	0.04 (-0.02 to 0.1)	NS	NS	Low (imprecision, medium risk of bias)
Magnesium	1	118	5.2	1.7	3.1 (0.3 to 29.0)	0.04 (-0.03 to 0.10)	NS	NS	Low (medium risk of bias, imprecision)

CI = confidence interval; NS = not significant; number needed to treat and number of attributable events were calculated for statistically significant differences);
RCT = randomized controlled trial
[a]Bold = significant differences at 95% confidence level when the 95% CI of attributable events does not include 0.

Table C. Evidence of migraine prevention in children: results from randomized controlled trials (RCTs)

Outcome	Active	Control	RCTs	Conclusion	Strength of Evidence (Reason for Lowering)
Complete cessation of headache attacks	Propranolol	Placebo	1	Propranolol was better than placebo in achieving complete cessation of migraine attacks.	Low (imprecision)
	Clonidine	Placebo	1	Clonidine was not better than placebo in achieving complete cessation of migraine attacks.	Low (imprecision)
	Sodium valproate	Propranolol	2	Sodium valproate and propranolol had no significant differences in complete cessation of headache attacks.	Low (medium risk of bias, imprecision)
Reduction by ≥50% in migraine attack frequency	Topiramate	Placebo	2	Topiramate, 50–200 mg/d, did not increase rate of reduction in migraine by ≥50%.	Moderate (medium risk of bias)
Reduction by ≥50% in migraine attack frequency	Divalproex sodium	Placebo	1	Divalproex sodium, 250–1,000 mg/d, did not increase rate of reduction in migraine by ≥50%.	Low (imprecision)
Reduction by ≥75% in migraine attack frequency	Propranolol	Placebo	1	Propranolol did not increase rate of reduction in migraine attacks by ≥75%.	Low (imprecision)
1–2 migraine frequency/month	Clonidine	Placebo	1	Clonidine did not increase rate of reduction in migraine.	Low (imprecision)
Reduction by ≥50% in migraine attack frequency	Sodium valproate	Propranolol	2	Sodium valproate and propranolol had no significant differences in reduction of migraine attack by ≥50% from baseline.	Low (medium risk of bias, imprecision)
Reduction by ≥50% in the headache index	Metoprolol	Progressive relaxation training + stress management	1	Metoprolol was less effective in reduction by ≥50% in headache index.	Low (unclear risk of bias, imprecision)
	Metoprolol	Cephalic vasomotor feedback + stress management	1	Metoprolol and cephalic vasomotor feedback + stress management had no significant differences in reduction by ≥50% In headache index.	Low (unclear risk of bias, imprecision)
Reduction in need for temporary drug therapy for single attacks	Clonidine	Placebo	1	Clonidine did not decrease use of drugs for acute migraine attacks.	Low (imprecision)
Improvement in Pediatric Migraine Disability Assessment Score	Topiramate	Sodium valproate	1	Topiramate and sodium valproate had no significant differences in Pediatric Migraine Disability Assessment Score.	Low (unclear risk of bias, imprecision)

RCT = randomized controlled trial

Off-Label Pharmacologic Agents: Antiepileptic Drugs

Topiramate
Topiramate, 50 to 200 mg/day, was no more effective than placebo in reducing monthly migraine attacks by ≥50 percent (two RCTs of 298 children, moderate-strength evidence). Topiramate increased the likelihood of ≥75 percent reduction in migraine days more often than placebo in a single double-blind RCT. Using this statistically significant risk difference, we estimated that 181 children (95% CI, 52 to 311) per 1,000 treated would experience a reduction of at least 75 percent in migraine days due to topiramate, 200 mg/day.

Divalproex Sodium
Divalproex sodium, 250 to 1,000 mg/day, was no more effective than placebo in reducing monthly migraine attacks by ≥50 percent in one RCT with low risk of bias (305 children, low-strength evidence). Divalproex sodium in doses of 250, 500, or 1,000 mg/day was no better than placebo in decreasing migraine days or decreasing use of drugs for acute attacks.

Off-Label Pharmacologic Agents: Beta Blockers
Propranolol resulted in a complete cessation of migraine attacks more often than placebo (one RCT of 28 children, low-strength evidence). We estimated that 713 children per 1,000 treated (95% CI, 452 to 974) would experience complete cessation of migraine attacks with propranolol. The same study separately examined the effectiveness of propranolol for reducing monthly migraine attacks by ≥50 percent and found no difference between propranolol and placebo.

Off-Label Pharmacologic Agents: Antidepressants
Trazodone was more effective than placebo for reducing frequency and duration of migraine attacks by 1.6 per month and reduced duration of migraine attacks by 8.2 hours per attack (one RCT of 40 children, low-strength evidence). No studies examined reducing monthly migraine attacks by ≥50 percent or other patient-centered outcomes.

Off-Label Pharmacologic Agents: Antiadrenergic Drugs
Clonidine was no more effective than placebo for reducing migraine duration or severity, or for reducing use of drugs for acute migraine attacks (one RCT of 57 children, low-strength evidence). No studies examined reducing monthly migraine attacks by ≥50 percent or other patient-centered outcomes.

Off-Label Pharmacologic Agents: Magnesium Oxide
A single RCT demonstrated no significant differences between magnesium oxide and placebo for reducing migraine frequency. Magnesium oxide reduced severity of migraine attacks relative to the placebo group. No studies examined reducing monthly migraine attacks by ≥50 percent or other patient-centered outcomes.

Key Question 1b. How do preventive pharmacologic treatments affect patient-centered and intermediate outcomes when compared with active pharmacologic treatments?

Limited evidence from individual RCTs suggested no differences for migraine prevention with examined drugs, including propranolol, valproate, and topiramate.

Two RCTs of 183 children examined the comparative effectiveness of sodium valproate versus propranolol (low-strength evidence) and found no significant differences between the drugs for complete cessation of headache attacks or ≥50 percent reduction from baseline migraine frequency. One RCT of 48 children examined the comparative effectiveness of topiramate versus sodium valproate (low-strength evidence) and found no difference in effects for migraine frequency, intensity, or duration, or for the Pediatric Migraine Disability Assessment Score.

Key Question 1c. How do preventive pharmacologic treatments affect patient-centered and intermediate outcomes when compared with active nonpharmacologic treatments?

Limited evidence from individual RCTs suggested that the beta blockers propranolol and metoprolol were less effective that nonpharmacologic treatments, including self-administered stress management and relaxation techniques. Two small RCTs compared drugs with active nonpharmacologic treatments. We concluded unclear risk of bias in both trials because the authors provided insufficient details about methodology.

One RCT examined the comparative effectiveness of metoprolol versus a nonpharmacologic intervention that combined stress management with either: (1) progressive relaxation training or (2) stress management training with cephalic vasomotor feedback, in which a photoplethysmograph was used to objectively measure brain blood volume changes. Stress management training included specific relaxation exercises in response to usual migraine triggers such as an intrusively noisy radio program or specific tasks demanding cognitive effort. This RCT found no significant differences between metoprolol and cephalic vasomotor feedback in the percentage of children who improved by ≥50 percent in the headache index (low-strength evidence).[26] In fact, metoprolol was less effective in preventing migraine or reducing migraine severity than stress management combined with progressive relaxation training.

One RCT of 33 children (low-strength evidence) compared the effectiveness of propranolol versus self-hypnosis. This trial found that migraine occurred more frequently with propranolol than with self-hypnosis.

Key Question 1d. How do preventive pharmacologic treatments combined with nondrug treatments affect patient-centered and intermediate outcomes when compared with pharmacologic treatments alone?

No studies compared combined treatments for migraine prevention with drugs alone.

Key Question 1e1. How might dosing regimens or duration of treatments influence the effects of the treatments on patient-centered outcomes?

Dose-response effects of preventive antiepileptic drugs in children were examined in four RCTs and one pooled analysis of three RCTs. All RCTs were double blind with low risk of bias. Higher doses of topiramate (100 to 200 mg/day) did not result in significantly better migraine prevention than lower doses. Higher doses of divalproex sodium (500 to 1,000 vs. 250 mg/day) did not result in significantly better migraine prevention than lower doses in a single RCT that examined this association.

Key Question 1e2. How might approaches to drug management (such as patient-care teams, integrated care, coordinated care, patient education, drug surveillance, or interactive drug monitoring) influence results?

Multidisciplinary drug management was more effective than usual care in preventing migraine in children and adolescents (one RCT), but the effect was not sustained at 6 months (one RCT of 68 children, low-strength evidence). The multimodal cognitive-behavioral training focused on stress management (perception of own stress symptoms, coping with stress), progressive relaxation techniques, cognitive restructuring (identification of dysfunctional cognitions regarding headache and self-assurance strategies such as being proactive and sensitive to one's own needs), and problem solving. The participants communicated through email with a multidisciplinary team of trial coordinators. The applied relaxation included progressive relaxation, cue-controlled relaxation (triggered by a key word or an image), and differential relaxation. We estimated that 310 children per 1,000 treated with multimodal cognitive-behavioral training would experience ≥50 percent reduction in migraine frequency (95-percent CI, 70 to 550). The effect, however, was not sustained at 6 months of followup. Migraine frequency and quality of life did not differ between Internet-based self-management versus an education program.

Key Question 2. What are the comparative harms from pharmacologic treatments for preventing migraine attacks in children?

Key Question 2a. What are the harms from preventive pharmacologic treatments when compared with placebo or no active treatment?

Overall, 10 randomized trials and one pooled analysis of 3 RCTs examined the safety of drugs for migraine prevention in children. The trials included 1,046 children. All RCTs were double blinded. Based on all risk-of-bias criteria, we concluded that six RCTs had low risk of bias and four had medium risk of bias. Sixteen nonrandomized studies reported harms of migraine preventive drugs in children. Evidence about treatment discontinuation due to adverse effects is presented in Table B.

Adverse Effects With Off-Label Pharmacologic Agents: Antiepileptic Drugs

Topiramate

Treatment discontinuation due to adverse effects was not more common with topiramate than with placebo in a pooled analysis of two RCTs (low-strength evidence). Topiramate increased risk of paresthesia, upper respiratory tract infection, and weight loss. Nonrandomized studies suggested that 19 percent of children discontinued topiramate treatments because of bothersome adverse effects.

We estimated from a single RCT that 260 children per 1,000 treated with topiramate (95% CI, 30 to 480) would experience adverse effects. Our pooled analysis of individual adverse effects demonstrated significant increase in risk of weight loss, paresthesia, and upper respiratory tract infection with topiramate. We estimated that for every 1,000 children treated with topiramate, 87 would experience unintended weight loss (95% CI, 24 to 150) and 105 would be diagnosed with upper respiratory tract infection (95% CI, 29 to 182). Rates of adverse effects did not differ among 50, 100, and 200 mg/day of topiramate.

Divalproex Sodium

Treatment discontinuation due to adverse effects was more common with 1,000 mg/day but not with 250 mg/day of divalproex sodium compared with placebo in one RCT (low-strength evidence). The analyses demonstrated that 80 children per 1,000 treated with divalproex sodium, 1,000 mg/day, would stop taking the drug due to intolerable adverse effects (95% CI, 9 to 151). Nonrandomized studies suggested that 84 percent of children experienced adverse effects with divalproex, and 17 percent discontinued treatment due to bothersome adverse effects.

Adverse Effects With Off-Label Pharmacologic Agents: Beta Blockers

A single RCT offered low-strength evidence that propranolol and placebo did not differ with regard to risk of any adverse effects.

Adverse Effects With Off-Label Pharmacologic Agents: Antidepressants

A single RCT with low risk of bias offered low-strength evidence that treatment discontinuation for any reason did not differ between the antidepressant trazodone and placebo in 40 children with migraine. One retrospective chart review demonstrated that, of 14 patients taking amitriptyline, 36 percent discontinued it at 16 weeks due to side effects.

Adverse Effects With Off-Label Pharmacologic Agents: Magnesium Oxide

A single RCT demonstrated no difference between magnesium oxide and placebo for risk of treatment discontinuation or for treatment discontinuation due to treatment failure or adverse effects.

Key Question 2b. What are the harms from preventive pharmacologic treatments when compared with other pharmacologic treatments?

A single RCT found no differences in adverse effects with topiramate and sodium valproate when administered for 12 weeks in 48 children with migraine.

Key Question 2c. How might approaches to drug management (such as patient-care teams, integrated care, coordinated care, patient education, drug surveillance, or interactive drug monitoring) improve safety of the treatments?

We found no studies that examined how drug management can improve safety of migraine preventive medications in children.

Key Question 3. Which characteristics of children predict the effectiveness and safety of pharmacologic treatments for preventing migraine attacks?

We found no studies that provided evidence for individualized treatment decisions for migraine prevention in children. No studies examined which characteristics of children might modify the effectiveness or safety of preventive drugs.

Discussion

Our comprehensive review identified limited evidence about benefits and harms of migraine preventive drugs in children. Limited evidence from individual RCTs suggested that only one drug, the beta blocker propranolol, prevented migraine more effectively than placebo (Table A).[27] Other examined drugs failed to prevent migraine in children, including the antiepileptic drugs topiramate and divalproex, the antiadrenergic drug clonidine, the antidepressant trazodone, and magnesium oxide. Moreover, we observed greater rates of treatment discontinuation due to adverse effects with divalproex sodium, 1,000 mg/day, and increased risk of weight loss, paresthesia, and respiratory tract infection with topiramate.

Previously published reviews also reported bothersome adverse effects with antiepileptic drugs in children with migraine[28,29] or epilepsy.[30] Off-label use of the antidepressant trazodone did not prevent migraine in children. We could not determine the effectiveness of other antidepressants for preventing migraine in children, nor could we determine whether adverse effects of antidepressants are similar when used for children with migraine compared to children with depression. We do know that antidepressants may increase risk of suicidal behavior in children and adolescents.[31] Use of off-label psychotropic drugs for migraine prevention could be justified in children with psychiatric comorbidity;[32] however, trials available for review did not report the presence of comorbid illnesses in enrolled patients.

Few included trials examined the seriousness or bothersomeness of harms with drugs. Clinicians who must make decisions about off-label drugs for children with migraine have very limited evidence about the balance between benefits and harms. Few clinical trials followed the recommendations from the Task Force on Adverse Events in Migraine Trials of the International Headache Society[33] when examining the potential harms of these drugs when used in children. Future fully powered trials involving children with migraine should examine the long-term safety of preventive drugs regardless of how investigators perceive the causality of the drugs on detected harms.

No studies sought to determine whether or how specific characteristics of children could predict the effectiveness or long-term safety of drugs for migraine prevention. Treatment effects may differ between children and adolescents, but published trials did not separately report results for age subgroups.

In head-to-head RCTs, metoprolol and propranolol were less effective than nonpharmacologic treatments. When both benefits and harms were analyzed, the nonpharmacologic treatments demonstrated better benefit-to-harm ratios than the drugs. Individualized multimodal drug management showed promising results.[34] Other complex disease-management interventions, including school-based psychological support or drug management, have both demonstrated positive results for treating acute headache attacks, but neither has been examined for migraine prevention.[35,36] RCTs have not yet examined other drug management interventions, including integrated care, coordinated care, patient education, drug surveillance, and interactive drug monitoring.

Evidence of drug benefits and harms was mostly low strength due to risk of bias and imprecise estimates from underpowered RCTs. The reporting quality of trials was poor; few trials provided detailed information about prior or concomitant treatments, comorbidities, family history, socioeconomic status, overuse of drugs for acute migraine treatment, or other important characteristics of the children studied. On average, the trials lasted 20 weeks. Given that these drugs are sometimes recommended for preventive use over very long periods, these trials did not provide sufficiently long-term evidence of benefits and harms. We could not determine the optimal duration of preventive drug treatment for children with migraine, nor could we determine the sustained benefits and harms of these treatments.

Key Messages

- Propranolol was more effective than placebo for preventing migraine in children, with no bothersome adverse effects that could lead to treatment discontinuation.
- Antiepileptics were no more effective than placebo in preventing migraine, but they resulted in increased risk of adverse effects.
- Internet-based self-management with multimodal cognitive training was better than education in preventing migraine in children and adolescents at 6 weeks but not 6 months of followup.
- Reporting quality was poor for studies involving children.

Limitations

Our review has limitations. We did not synthesize the evidence for flunarizine because the FDA has not approved it; however, this drug has been shown in RCTs to be effective in preventing migraines in children. One RCT with low risk of bias suggested that flunarizine resulted in ≥50 percent reduction in migraine attacks in 500 children per 1,000 treated (95% CI, 260 to 740). A comprehensive review of nonpharmacologic treatments was beyond our scope.

Our comprehensive literature search of several databases, trial registries, and FDA reviews detected a very low publication rate of registered completed clinical trials involving children. We could not determine why the studies were not published. We assumed publication bias but did not contact the investigators of completed trials for unpublished data. We did request additional data from the sponsors of completed trials, but we received few responses. Thus, we know neither the results from unpublished trials nor how many unregistered studies have been conducted and never published. We relied on reported information and did not contact study authors for additional details (such as trial design, execution, or poorly reported results we could not reproduce).

Research Gaps

Our report offers insights for future research. Future trials should be conducted according to the recently published Standards for Research in Child Health.[37] RCTs should examine the comparative effectiveness of multimodal drug and disease management; long-term benefits, safety, and adherence with preventive treatments; and the role of children's characteristics that could modify benefits and harms of preventive drugs.

Future studies should also specifically examine the effects and risks of off-label drug use for migraine prevention in children. Randomized trials have examined only a few pharmacologic agents. However, practicing clinicians may prescribe many off-label drugs to treat children, and little is known about the comparative effectiveness or safety of the drug classes used. Large observational studies, including the American Migraine Prevalence and Prevention Study, relied on self-reported use of preventive medications and did not assess exact drug use or effectiveness.[5] The few available studies of off-label drug use in children show that 5 percent of all antiepileptic drug prescriptions were for migraine.[38] The National Ambulatory Medical Care Surveys (NAMCS) from 2001 to 2004 demonstrated that 62 percent of all outpatient pediatric visits included off-label prescriptions, 86 percent of which were for pain.[39] European studies demonstrated that overall about 30 percent of hospitalized children[40] and 40 percent of children in outpatient settings received off-label drug prescriptions.[41] European observational studies found a significantly higher risk of adverse effects with off-label drugs than other drugs and concluded that there is an improper balance of benefits and risks with off-label drugs in pediatric patients.[41]

As a first step, the comparative effectiveness and safety of off-label drugs used for migraine prevention in children should be examined by analyzing administrative databases. Such analyses could shed light on practice patterns in migraine prevention and provide insight into the comparative effectiveness of preventive drugs for reducing visits to emergency rooms. Based on these analyses, RCTs could be designed to examine the drugs found to have the most favorable ratios of benefits to harms.

Existing clinical research policy does not guarantee the availability of results from all studies involving children. Results are unavailable for more than half of the studies involving children, suggesting a substantial publication bias.[42] Registration and posting of results on ClinicalTrials.gov should be mandatory for all studies involving children including children with migraine.[42]

References

1. Goadsby PJ, Raskin NH. Headache. In: Fauci AS, Braunwald E, Kasper DL, et al., eds. Harrison's Principles of Internal Medicine. 17th ed. New York: The McGraw-Hill Companies; 2008:chapter 15.

2. Headache Classification Subcommittee of the International Headache Society. The International Classification of Headache Disorders: 2nd edition. Cephalalgia. 2004;24(Suppl 1):9-160. PMID: 14979299.

3. Silberstein SD. Preventive migraine treatment. Neurol Clin. 2009 May;27(2):429-43. PMID: 19289224.

4. Solomon GD, Santanello N. Impact of migraine and migraine therapy on productivity and quality of life. Neurology. 2000;55(9 Suppl 2):S29-35. PMID: 11089517.

5. Diamond S, Bigal ME, Silberstein S, et al. Patterns of diagnosis and acute and preventive treatment for migraine in the United States: results from the American Migraine Prevalence and Prevention study. Headache. 2007 Mar;47(3):355-63. PMID: 17371352.

6. Lipton RB, Scher AI, Kolodner K, et al. Migraine in the United States: epidemiology and patterns of health care use. Neurology. 2002 Mar 26;58(6):885-94. PMID: 11914403.

7. Bigal ME, Lipton RB, Winner P, et al. Migraine in adolescents: association with socioeconomic status and family history. Neurology. 2007 Jul 3;69(1):16-25. PMID: 17606878.

8. Hernandez-Latorre MA, Roig M. Natural history of migraine in childhood. Cephalalgia. 2000 Jul;20(6):573-9. PMID: 11075841.

9. Lipton RB, Manack A, Ricci JA, et al. Prevalence and burden of chronic migraine in adolescents: results of the Chronic Daily Headache in Adolescents Study (C-dAS). Headache. 2011 May;51(5):693-706. PMID: 21521206.

10. Lipton RB, Stewart WF, Diamond S, et al. Prevalence and burden of migraine in the United States: data from the American Migraine Study II. Headache. 2001 Jul-Aug;41(7):646-57. PMID: 11554952.

11. Fraguas D, Merchan-Naranjo J, Laita P, et al. Metabolic and hormonal side effects in children and adolescents treated with second-generation antipsychotics. J Clin Psychiatry. 2008 Jul;69(7):1166-75. PMID: 18588363.

12. Correll CU, Carlson HE. Endocrine and metabolic adverse effects of psychotropic medications in children and adolescents. J Am Acad Child Adolesc Psychiatry. 2006 Jul;45(7):771-91. PMID: 16832314.

13. Pappagallo M, Silva R. The effect of atypical antipsychotic agents on prolactin levels in children and adolescents. J Child Adolesc Psychopharmacol. 2004 Fall;14(3):359-71. PMID: 15650493.

14. Kumra S, Oberstar JV, Sikich L, et al. Efficacy and tolerability of second-generation antipsychotics in children and adolescents with schizophrenia. Schizophr Bull. 2008 Jan;34(1):60-71. PMID: 17923452.

15. Dubois D. Toxicology and overdose of atypical antipsychotic medications in children: does newer necessarily mean safer? Curr Opin Pediatr. 2005 Apr;17(2):227-33. PMID: 15800418.

16. Whitlock EP, Lopez SA, Chang S, et al. AHRQ series paper 3: identifying, selecting, and refining topics for comparative effectiveness systematic reviews: AHRQ and the effective health-care program. J Clin Epidemiol. 2010 May;63(5):491-501. PMID: 19540721.

17. Slutsky J, Atkins D, Chang S, et al. Comparing medical interventions: AHRQ and the Effective Health Care Program. Methods Guide for Effectiveness and Comparative Effectiveness Reviews. AHRQ Publication No. 10(11)-EHC063-EF. Rockville, MD: Agency for Healthcare Research and Quality; March 2011. Chapters available at www.effectivehealthcare.ahrq.gov.

18. Helfand M, Balshem H. Principles in developing and applying guidance. Methods Guide for Effectiveness and Comparative Effectiveness Reviews. AHRQ Publication No. 10(11)-EHC063-EF. Rockville, MD: Agency for Healthcare Research and Quality; March 2011. Chapters available at www.effectivehealthcare.ahrq.gov. PMID: 21433405.

19. Liberati A, Altman DG, Tetzlaff J, et al. The PRISMA statement for reporting systematic reviews and meta-analyses of studies that evaluate health care interventions: explanation and elaboration. Ann Intern Med. 2009 Aug 18;151(4):W65-94. PMID: 19622512.

20. Norris S, Atkins D, Bruening W, et al. Selecting observational studies for comparing medical interventions. Methods Guide for Effectiveness and Comparative Reviews. AHRQ Publication No. 10(11)-EHC063-EF. Rockville, MD: Agency for Healthcare Research and Quality. March 2011:56-68:chapter 4. Chapters available at: www.effectivehealthcare.ahrq.gov.

21. Higgins J, Green S, eds. Cochrane Handbook for Systematic Reviews of Interventions. Version 5.1.0. London: The Cochrane Collaboration; 2011.

22. Olesen J, Bousser MG, Diener HC, et al. New appendix criteria open for a broader concept of chronic migraine. Cephalalgia. 2006 Jun;26(6):742-6. PMID: 16686915.

23. Owens DK, Lohr KN, Atkins D, et al. AHRQ series paper 5: grading the strength of a body of evidence when comparing medical interventions-Agency for Healthcare Research and Quality and the Effective Health-Care Program. J Clin Epidemiol. 2010 May;63(5):513-23. PMID: 19595577.

24. Guyatt G, Oxman AD, Kunz R, et al. GRADE guidelines 6. Rating the quality of evidence-imprecision. J Clin Epidemiol. 2011 Dec;64(12):1283-93. Epub 2011 Aug 11. PMID: 21839614.

25. Atkins D, Chang SM, Gartlehner G, et al. Assessing applicability when comparing medical interventions: AHRQ and the Effective Health Care Program. J Clin Epidemiol. 2011 Nov;64(11):1198-207. PMID: 21463926.

26. Sartory G, Muller B, Metsch J, et al. A comparison of psychological and pharmacological treatment of pediatric migraine. Behav Res Ther. 1998 Dec;36(12):1155-70. PMID: 9745800.

27. Victor S, Ryan SW. Drugs for preventing migraine headaches in children. Cochrane Database Syst Rev. 2003;(4):CD002761. PMID: 14583952.

28. Jayapal S, Maheshwari N. Question 3. Topiramate for chronic migraine in children. Arch Dis Child. 2011 Mar;96(3):318-21. PMID: 21317129.

29. Damen L, Bruijn J, Verhagen AP, et al. Prophylactic treatment of migraine in children. Part 2. A systematic review of pharmacological trials. Cephalalgia. 2006 May;26(5):497-505. PMID: 16674757.

30. Connock M, Frew E, Evans BW, et al. The clinical effectiveness and cost-effectiveness of newer drugs for children with epilepsy. A systematic review. Health Technol Assess. 2006 Mar;10(7):iii, ix-118. PMID: 16545206.

31. Bridge JA, Iyengar S, Salary CB, et al. Clinical response and risk for reported suicidal ideation and suicide attempts in pediatric antidepressant treatment: a meta-analysis of randomized controlled trials. JAMA. 2007 Apr 18;297(15):1683-96. PMID: 17440145.

32. Breslau N. Psychiatric comorbidity in migraine. Cephalalgia. 1998 Aug;18(Suppl 22):56-8; discussion 8-61. PMID: 9793713.

33. Tfelt-Hansen P, Bjarnason NH, Dahlof C, et al. Evaluation and registration of adverse events in clinical drug trials in migraine. Cephalalgia. 2008 Jul;28(7):683-8. PMID: 18498392.

34. Trautmann E, Kroner-Herwig B. A randomized controlled trial of Internet-based self-help training for recurrent headache in childhood and adolescence. Behav Res Ther. 2010 Jan;48(1):28-37. PMID: 19782343.

35. Larsson B, Carlsson J, Fichtel A, et al. Relaxation treatment of adolescent headache sufferers: results from a school-based replication series. Headache. 2005 Jun;45(6):692-704. PMID: 15953302.

36. Fichtel A, Larsson B. Relaxation treatment administered by school nurses to adolescents with recurrent headaches. Headache. 2004 Jun;44(6):545-54. PMID: 15186298.

37. Hartling L, Wittmeier KDM, Caldwell P, et al. StaR child health: developing evidence-based guidance for the design, conduct, and reporting of pediatric trials. Pediatrics. 2012 June 1;129(Suppl 3):S112-S7.

38. van de Vrie-Hoekstra NW, de Vries TW, van den Berg PB, et al. Antiepileptic drug utilization in children from 1997-2005--a study from the Netherlands. Eur J Clin Pharmacol. 2008 Oct;64(10):1013-20. PMID: 18618103.

39. Bazzano AT, Mangione-Smith R, Schonlau M, et al. Off-label prescribing to children in the United States outpatient setting. Acad Pediatr. 2009 Mar-Apr;9(2):81-8. PMID: 19329098.

40. Choonara I, Conroy S. Unlicensed and off-label drug use in children: implications for safety. Drug Safety. 2002;25(1):1-5. PMID: 11820908.

41. Horen B, Montastruc JL, Lapeyre-Mestre M. Adverse drug reactions and off-label drug use in paediatric outpatients. Br J Clin Pharmacol. 2002 Dec;54(6):665-70. PMID: 12492616.

42. Shamliyan T, Kane RL. Clinical research involving children: registration, completeness, and publication. Pediatrics. 2012 May;129(5):e1291-300. PMID: 22529271.

Introduction

In the United States, migraine affects a significant number of children: 5 percent of boys[1,2] and 7.7 percent of girls (Table 1).[3,4] The American Migraine Prevalence and Prevention study of 32,015 adolescents found that childhood migraine is more prevalent in lower income families.[3] The same study reported that among adolescents, migraine is more prevalent in Whites than African Americans.[3]

Table 1. Prevalence of migraine headache through childhood[5]

	3–7 Years of Age	7–11 Years of Age	15 Years of Age
Prevalence	1.2%–3.2%	4%–11%	8%–23%
Ratio by Sex	Boys > girls	Boys = girls	Girls > boys

According to the International Classification of Headache Disorders (second edition) (ICHD-II), migraine is a common disabling primary headache disorder manifesting in attacks that last from 4 to 72 hours.[6,7] Migraine pain results primarily from increased activity of several agents that regulate blood vessels and sensory function of the brain.[6] Migraine headaches range from moderate to very severe[8] and are sometimes debilitating.

Migraine frequency is classified as either episodic or chronic based on the number of monthly migraine days[7] (episodic is <15 days, and chronic is ≥15 days). Chronic migraine affects 2 percent of children and adolescents (Table 2).[9]

Table 2. Chronic migraine prevalence rates, from the Chronic Daily Headache in Adolescents Study (C-dAS)*

Characteristic	Population Category	Prevalence[†]	Prevalence[‡]
All adolescents	12-17	0.79 (0.00 to 1.70)	1.75 (0.62 to 2.89)
Age, years	12-13	0.09 (0.00 to 0.19)	0.30 (0.12 to 0.48)
Age, years	14-15	0.22 (0.06 to 0.38)	1.04 (0.52 to 1.57)
Age, years	16-17	2.02 (0.00 to 4.71)	3.86 (0.45 to 7.26)
Sex	Male	0.15 (0.05 to 0.26)	0.55 (0.22 to 0.88)
Sex	Female	1.39 (0 to 2.87)	3.11 (0.70 to 5.53)

ICHD-IIR = International Classification of Headache Disorders, second edition, revised
*Prevalence estimates adjusted for nonresponse/noncoverage and benchmarked to U.S. Census data[9].
[†]Adapted ICHD-IIR criteria (>15 headache days per month, >8 days of ICHD-II pediatric migraine, or most frequent headache medication was a triptan or ergot; >5 lifetime attacks of ICHD-II pediatric migraine; and no medication overuse).
[‡]Adapted ICHD-IIR criteria used for CM and including individuals with (+) and without (-) medication overuse.

Migraine is further classified by whether or not it involves aura. Migraine with aura is characterized by episodes of intense disabling headache with visual symptoms or distortions that begin gradually and last for several minutes.[5] Approximately 15 to 30 percent of children and adolescents with migraine experience aura.[5] The diagnostic criteria for migraine with aura include brief duration (1 to 72 hours), bilateral or bifrontal location (age <15 years), and the inference of photophobia and phonophobia by behavioral response rather than verbal report.[5] The most frequent forms of aura are binocular visual impairment with scotoma (77 percent), distortion or hallucinations (16 percent), and monocular visual impairment or scotoma (7 percent).[5] Other accompanying symptoms may include photophobia (excessive sensitivity to light), phonophobia (fear of loud sounds), osmophobia (hypersensitivity to smells), nausea, or vomiting.[8]

Migraine significantly affects children's physical, psychological, and social well-being. It can impose serious lifestyle restrictions.[9] Indeed, the majority of adolescents with chronic migraine have migraine-related disability.[9] Yet, according to the Chronic Daily Headache in

Adolescents Study, fewer than half of adolescents with chronic migraine had visited a healthcare provider. Fewer than one in five had taken medications to prevent headaches during the previous month.[9]

Prospective epidemiologic studies that followed children with migraine for decades demonstrated that around 20 percent became migraine free before the age of 25 (boys significantly more often than girls).[10,11] However, more than half of children with migraine experienced attacks through middle and older age.[10]

Childhood migraine, whether chronic or episodic, can have a serious detrimental impact on daily life. Approximately 31 percent of children with migraine missed at least 1 day of school in the previous 3 months because of the condition.[12] Childhood migraine has also been shown to impair learning and school productivity by ≥50 percent.[12] Many children with frequent or severe attacks need treatment, which may aim either to ameliorate acute attacks or to prevent attacks. Drugs used to treat acute migraine attacks in children include nonsteroid anti-inflammatory agents, triptans, and antiepileptics.[13] Our review focuses on preventive pharmacologic treatments for childhood migraine.

Preventive medications are presumed to address the pathophysiology of migraine.[14,15] The four drugs approved by the U.S. Food and Drug Administration (FDA) for migraine prevention in adults come from different drug classes and include propranolol, timolol, topiramate, and divalproex sodium.[16] The FDA has approved no drugs for migraine prevention in children; therefore, pediatricians prescribe either drugs approved for adults or off-label drugs (approved for clinical conditions other than migraine prevention).[16,17] These drug classes cause common and serious adverse effects, including metabolic and hormonal abnormalities.[18-22] Therefore, migraine preventive drug choices should be based on efficacy and safety of the available drugs, whether approved for adults or used off label.[23-30]

Preventive treatment aims to eliminate headache pain.[23,24,31] Often, however, some pain persists; therefore, treatment success is usually defined by a decrease in migraine frequency by ≥50 percent after 3 months.[8] In addition to pain relief, preventive drugs can also decrease severity of migraine attacks and reduce restrictions in daily activities and schooling.[32,33] Some guidelines recommend preventive treatments for patients who have five or more migraine attacks per month,[6] while others suggest it for those who experience a headache on most days of the month.[25,34,35] No studies have examined outcomes of preventive treatments for long-term migraine frequency and adverse effects.[8]

Gaps remain in the published literature on preventive treatments for migraine in children. Published systematic reviews have focused on the efficacy of specific drugs rather than comparative effectiveness of all available pharmacologic and nonpharmacologic treatments, including multidisciplinary migraine management programs. Furthermore, evidence syntheses have neither consistently assessed risk of bias in individual studies nor evaluated strength of evidence about benefits and harms with available treatments.

Our review focuses on the comparative effectiveness and safety of drugs for preventing migraine attacks in children in ambulatory care settings; our results will help inform related treatment recommendations.

Topic Refinement and Review Protocol

During the topic refinement stage, we solicited input from Key Informants representing medical professional societies/clinicians in the areas of neurology, primary care, consumers, scientific experts, and payers, to help define the Key Questions (KQs).[36] The KQs were then posted for public comment for 4 weeks from April 12, 2012, to May 10, 2012, and the comments received were considered in the development of the research protocol. We next convened a Technical Expert Panel (TEP) comprising clinical, content, and methodological experts to provide input in defining populations, interventions, comparisons, and outcomes and in identifying particular studies or databases to search. The Key Informants and members of the TEP were required to disclose any financial conflicts of interest greater than $10,000 and any other relevant business or professional conflicts. Any potential conflicts of interest were balanced or mitigated. Neither Key Informants nor members of the TEP performed analysis of any kind, nor did any of them contribute to the writing of this report. Members of the TEP were invited to provide feedback on an initial draft of the review protocol, which was then refined based on their input, reviewed by AHRQ, and posted for public access at the AHRQ Effective Health Care Website.

We chose not to synthesize studies of flunarizine, because it lacks FDA approval. Efficacy of nonpharmacologic preventive treatments was beyond our scope. We conducted a comprehensive literature review following the principles in the Methods Guide for Effectiveness and Comparative Effectiveness Reviews (hereafter Methods Guide) developed by the Agency for Healthcare Research and Quality (AHRQ) Evidence-based Practice Center (EPC) Program[37,38] and PRISMA guidelines (protocol registration number is CRD42011001858, available at http://www.crd.york.ac.uk/prospero/display_record.asp?ID=CRD42011001858).[39]

Key Questions

Key Question 1. What is the efficacy and comparative effectiveness of pharmacologic treatments for preventing migraine attacks in children?

   a. How do preventive pharmacologic treatments affect patient-centered and intermediate outcomes when compared to placebo or no active treatment?

   b. How do preventive pharmacologic treatments affect patient-centered and intermediate outcomes when compared to active pharmacologic treatments?

   c. How do preventive pharmacologic treatments affect patient-centered and intermediate outcomes when compared to active nonpharmacologic treatments?

   d. How do preventive pharmacologic treatments combined with nondrug treatments affect patient-centered and intermediate outcomes when compared to pharmacologic treatments alone?

   e. How might dosing regimens or duration of treatments influence the effects of the treatments on patient-centered outcomes? How might approaches to drug management (such as patient care teams, integrated care, coordinated care, patient education, drug surveillance, or interactive drug monitoring) influence results?

Key Question 2. What are the comparative harms from pharmacologic treatments for preventing migraine attacks in children?

  a. What are the harms from preventive pharmacologic treatments when compared to placebo or no active treatment?
  b. What are the harms from preventive pharmacologic treatments when compared to active pharmacologic treatments?
  c. How might approaches to drug management (such as patient care teams, integrated care, coordinated care, patient education, drug surveillance, or interactive drug monitoring) improve safety of the treatments?

Key Question 3. Which characteristics of children predict the effectiveness and safety of pharmacologic treatments for preventing migraine attacks?

Methods

We followed an a priori research protocol that we developed with the clinical and methodological input of the TEP. The protocol followed the Effective Health Care Program's "Methods Guide for Effectiveness and Comparative Effectiveness Reviews."

Literature Search Strategy

We searched for published studies in several databases, including MEDLINE® (via Ovid and PubMed®), the Cochrane Library, and the SCIRUS bibliographic database. We searched the FDA Web site for medical and statistical reviews of the eligible drugs. We searched clinical trial registries including ClinicalTrials.gov and the World Health Organization International Clinical Trials Registry to find ongoing, completed, and published trials of migraine prevention. We requested Scientific Information Packets from appropriate manufacturers (shown in Appendix A) per usual procedures. To find relevant unpublished studies, we reviewed the reference lists of identified guidelines, textbooks, and systematic reviews. We searched for the studies published in English up to May 20, 2012. We did not contact the investigators of the primary studies for missing data or clarifications.

The EPC developed a search strategy based on relevant medical subject heading (MeSH®) terms, text words, and weighted word-frequency algorithms to identify related articles. Exact search strategies can be found in Appendix A. Ongoing completed studies are shown in Appendix B.

Searches for relevant literature involved several steps: (1) evaluating previously published systematic reviews,[40] (2) conducting a comprehensive literature search in the above databases to retrieve identified references, (3) screening abstracts against the inclusion/exclusion criteria, and (4) reviewing full-text articles of eligible studies to determine potential inclusion in the synthesis.

Inclusion Criteria

We defined the target population, eligible preventive treatments, outcomes, time, and setting following the PICOTS framework (Population, Intervention, Comparator, Outcome, Timing, and Setting) (Appendix C Analytical framework). We defined the target population as community-dwelling children with episodic migraine, chronic daily headache, or chronic migraine defined according to criteria set by the International Headache Society.[25] In order to synthesize the evidence from trials published before the most recent International Headache Society diagnostic criteria for migraine, we included trials that used previous definitions of chronic daily headache.

We formulated a list of eligible interventions after discussions with key informants and technical experts, and after consideration of public comments. Eligible comparators included pharmacologic, nonpharmacologic, and combined preventive treatments. We defined eligible intermediate and patient-centered outcomes (presented in the analytical framework, Figure 1).

Our inclusion criteria were:

1. Original epidemiologic studies that aimed to examine preventive pharmacologic treatments for migraine.
2. Publication in English.
3. Target population of community-dwelling children with episodic migraine, chronic daily headache, or chronic migraine defined according to International Headache Society criteria for chronic migraine.[25]

4. Eligible intermediate and patient-centered outcomes as listed in the analytical framework (Figure 1).

We reviewed original clinical studies that included children with migraine, comorbid headache disorders, or tension headache as long as they examined prevention of migraine. Episodic or chronic migraine as defined by the Headache Classification Committee of the International Headache Society[25] does not include migraine variants or migraine equivalents with atypical symptomatic pain in regions other than the head.[7,42] Therefore, we exclude these studies.

Exclusion Criteria

1. Studies of treatments aimed at acute migraine attacks.
2. Studies that involved patients with migraine variants, such as basilar migraine, childhood periodic syndromes, retinal migraine, complicated migraines, and ophthalmoplegic migraine, hospitalized patients, or patients in emergency rooms.[7,42,43] We also excluded hemiplegic migraine, a pathophysiologically distinct disorder with its own classification.[43]
3. Studies of short-term prevention of migraine, including menstrual migraines.
4. Studies that included some pediatric patients with migraine but did not separately report those outcomes.
5. Studies that involved surgical treatments for migraine.
6. Preclinical pharmacokinetic studies of eligible drugs; studies that examined the pathophysiology of migraine reporting instrumental measurements or biochemical outcomes.
7. Studies that did not test the associative hypotheses.
8. Studies that examined eligible drugs on populations with other diseases.
9. Studies evaluating the efficacy of nonpharmacologic treatments or economic outcomes were beyond the scope of this review.

Study Selection

We followed the AHRQ Methods Guide to select evidence from controlled trials and observational studies.[44] Three investigators independently determined study eligibility resolving disagreement in discussions until consensus was achieved, as recommended by the "Cochrane Handbook for Systematic Reviews of Interventions."[45] To assess treatment benefits, we included randomized controlled trials (RCTs). To assess treatment harms, we included all available evidence from RCTs and observational studies.[44,46] We defined harms as a totality of all possible adverse consequences of an intervention.[46] We analyzed harms regardless of how authors perceived causality of treatments.

Figure 1. Analytical framework[37,38,41]

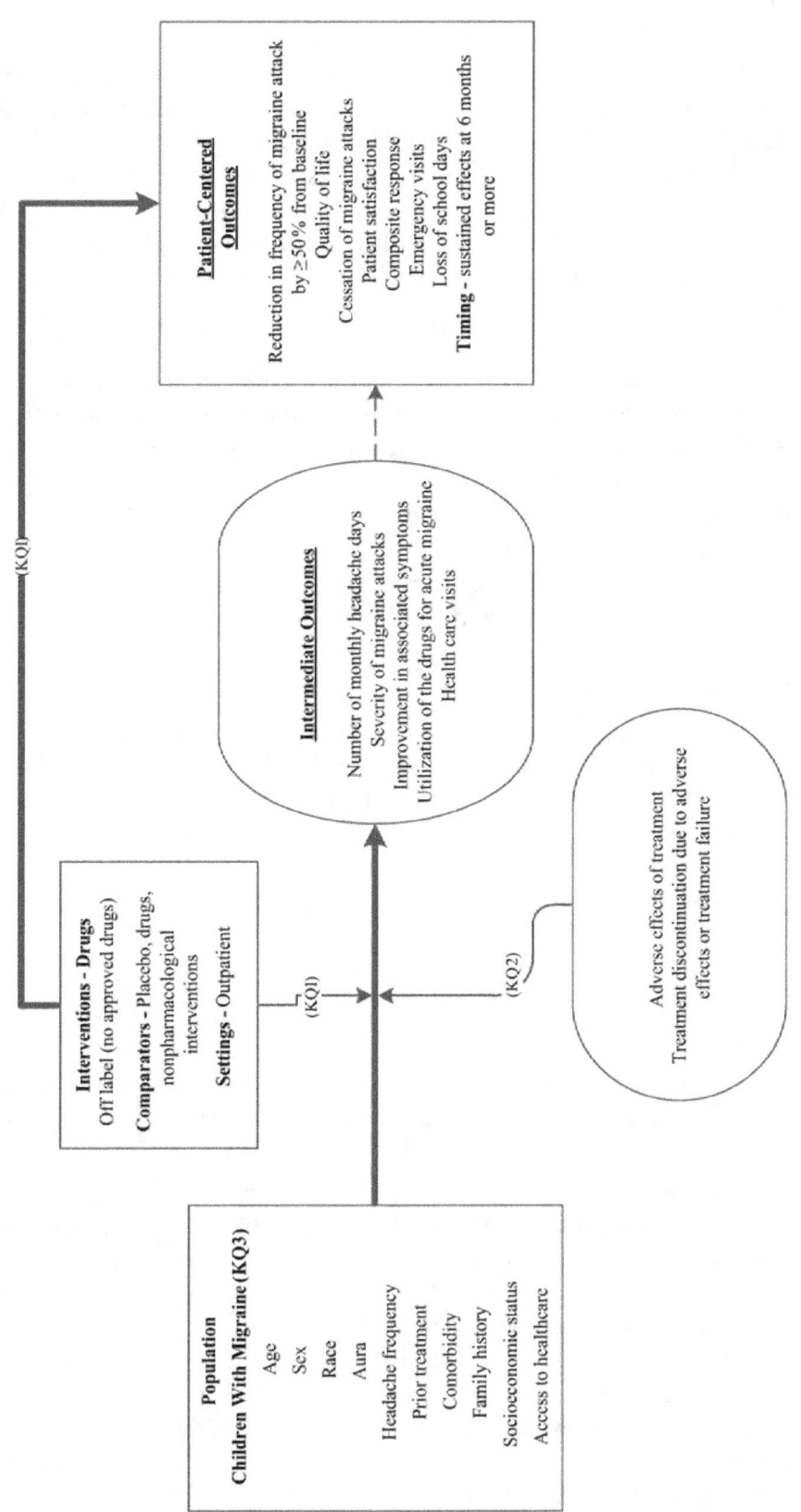

KQ = Key Question
Key Question 1: What is the efficacy and comparative effectiveness of pharmacologic treatments for preventing migraine attacks in children?
Key Question 2: What are the comparative harms from pharmacologic treatments for preventing migraine attacks in children?
Key Question 3: Which characteristics of children predict the effectiveness and safety of pharmacologic treatments for preventing migraine attacks?

Data Extraction

Researchers used standardized forms to extract data (available at https://netfiles.umn.edu/xythoswfs/webui/_xy-21041343_1-t_zdhvSpvy). For each trial, one reviewer abstracted an article and a second reviewer checked the abstracted data for accuracy. We assessed errors by comparing established ranges for each variable with data charts from the original articles. Detected discrepancies were discussed. We abstracted the information relevant to the PICOTS framework. We abstracted minimum datasets to reproduce the results presented by the authors. For categorical variables, we abstracted the number of events among treatment groups to calculate rates, relative risk, and absolute risk differences. We abstracted means and standard deviations of continuous variables to calculate mean differences with a 95% confidence interval (CI).

For RCTs in the quantitative analysis set, we abstracted the number randomized to each treatment group as the denominator to calculate estimates by applying intention-to-treat principles. We abstracted the time when the outcomes were assessed as weeks from randomization and the time of followup after treatments.

We abstracted inclusion and exclusion criteria, drug regimen and doses, and patient characteristics including demographics, baseline frequency, severity, and prior treatment status as factors that could modify treatment effects. We abstracted migraine definitions used in each study. We abstracted sponsorship of the studies and conflict of interest by the authors.

Risk of Bias Assessment

We evaluated the risk of bias in individual studies according to recommendations from the "Cochrane Handbook for Systematic Reviews of Interventions."[45] First, we classified the study design as interventional (an RCT, a nonrandomized controlled clinical trial, or a nonrandomized uncontrolled clinical trial) or observational (cohort or case-control studies, cross-sectional studies, or case series).

Then, using the criteria from the Cochrane risk of bias tool in interventional studies,[47] we evaluated:

- Random allocation of the subjects to the treatment groups.
- Masking of the treatment status.
- Adequacy of allocation concealment.
- Adequacy of randomization according to baseline similarity of the subjects in treatment groups by demographics, migraine frequency and severity, and response to previous treatments.
- Intention-to-treat principles.
- Selective outcome reporting when compared to the posted protocols (when trials were registered) or methods section in the articles.

We assumed a low risk of bias when RCTs met all the risk of bias criteria; a medium risk of bias if at least one risk of bias criterion was not met; and a high risk of bias if two or more risk of bias criteria were not met. We concluded an unknown risk of bias for the studies with poorly reported risk of bias criteria. Since all outcomes in the review are self-reported, masking of outcome assessment was not essential in evaluating risk of bias, but masking of treatment was. Masking of treatment status was not feasible for RCTs that examined nondrug therapies as comparators. Therefore, for these RCTs we did not include masking in our risk of bias assessments. We appraised risk of bias in nonrandomized studies according to selection, attrition, and detection biases.[48]

We evaluated disclosure of conflict of interest by the authors of individual studies and funding sources but did not use this information to downgrade quality of individual studies.

Data Synthesis

We summarized the results into evidence tables. We focused on the patient-centered outcomes of reduction in migraine attacks by $\geq$50 percent from baseline, quality of life, patient satisfaction, and composite outcomes that included migraine frequency and severity. We incorporated risk of bias in individual studies into the synthesis of evidence by using individual risk of bias criteria rather than a global score or a ranking category of overall risk of bias.[49,50] Our evidence synthesis about comparative benefits and safety with drugs from individual RCTs was restricted to studies with low or medium risk of bias.[23]

We synthesized the evidence according to population characteristics that could modify treatment effects, including age, sex, and race; duration of migraine; baseline frequency and severity of acute migraine attacks; presence of aura; previous drug treatments; history of drug overuse; and other patient characteristics described in the PICOTS framework. We addressed the role of comorbidities and concomitant treatments in association with patient-centered outcomes. When possible, based on the reporting in original studies, we conducted subgroup and sensitivity analyses according to patient characteristics, drug dose, and timing of followup.

Using Meta-Analyst[51] and STATA[®52] software, we calculated the relative risk and absolute risk difference from the abstracted events and the mean differences in continuous variables from the reported means and standard deviations. We evaluated statistical significance at a 95% confidence level.

We analyzed adjusted relative risk from observational studies that examined the association between treatments and patient-centered outcomes. We used correction coefficients (0.5 as a default in statistical software) and enforced intention to treat as recommended calculations for missing data.[45] We synthesized sparse data (defined as rates less than 2 percent) on adverse effects of the drugs using Peto odds ratio[53] and arcsine transformed absolute risk.[51,54-57] We evaluated the robustness of adverse effects estimates by comparing the results from described statistical models.

Pooling criteria for Key Questions 1 and 2 included the same active drug treatments and comparators and the same definitions of the outcomes.

For continuous outcomes we calculated mean difference and Cohen standardized mean differences for different continuous measures of the same outcome. To address clinical importance of the changes in continuous outcomes we also calculated means ratio.[58] The means ratios clarified clinical interpretations of the differences in means.

We tested consistency in the results by comparing the direction and strength of the association,[59] and we assessed heterogeneity in results with Chi-square and I-square tests.[60,61] We explored heterogeneity with meta-regression and sensitivity analysis, reporting the results from random effects models only.[62] Using the random effects model, we incorporated into the pooled analysis any differences between trials in patient populations, baseline rates of the outcomes, dosage of drugs, and other factors.[53] We explored heterogeneity by risk of bias criteria, disclosed conflicts of interest, study sponsorship, dose and duration of drug treatments, time of followup, inclusion of minorities, and other patient characteristics described above. To avoid ecological fallacy, we did not use patient level variables (for example, mean age or body mass index) in meta-regression.[62] We focused on direct comparisons and synthesized evidence from head-to-head comparative effectiveness studies. We did not attempt to conduct network meta-analysis of sparse data.

The number needed to treat to achieve one event of a patient-centered outcome was calculated as the reciprocal of statistically significant absolute risk differences (ARD) in rates of outcome events in the active and control groups.[52,63] We calculated means and 95% CIs for the number needed to treat as reciprocal of pooled ARD when ARD is significant.[64] The number of avoided or excess events (respectively) per population of 1,000 is the difference between the two events rates multiplied by 1,000. We calculated Bayesian odds ratios[51,57] with 95% credible intervals. All calculations were performed at a 95% confidence level.

Grading the Evidence for Each Key Question

We assessed strength of evidence according to risk of bias, consistency, directness, and precision for each patient-centered outcome including 100 percent or ≥50 percent reduction in monthly migraine frequency, patient global assessment of treatment success, and rates of clinically important improvement in migraine-related disability and quality of life, and treatment discontinuation due to harms.[59] We defined treatment effect estimates as precise when pooled estimates had reasonably narrow 95% CIs, or pooled sample had ≥300 events.[65] We did not include justification of the sample size into grading of the evidence, nor did we conduct *post hoc* statistical power analysis.

We defined reporting bias as publication bias, selective outcomes reporting, and multiple publication bias. We did not perform formal statistical tests to quantify the biases.[66]

In assessing strength of evidence, we also looked at dose-response association and strength of association in nonrandomized studies. We evaluated the strength of the association, defining a priori as a large effect when relative risk was >2 or <0.5 and a very large effect when relative risk was >5 or <0.2.[45] We defined low magnitude of effect when the relative risk was significant but <2.

We defined a high strength of evidence on the basis of consistent findings from well-designed RCTs (Table 3). We downgraded strength of evidence to moderate if at least one of the four strength of evidence criteria (risk of bias, directness, consistency, and precision) was not met; for example, the studies had medium risk of bias or the results were not consistent or precise. We downgraded strength of evidence to low if two or more criteria were not met. We assigned a low level of evidence to nonrandomized studies and upgraded strength of evidence for strong or dose-response associations. We defined evidence as insufficient when a single study with high risk of bias examined treatment effects or associations. To better inform decisionmaking, our presentation of results includes estimates of treatment effects and our strength of evidence evaluations.[67] Because insufficient evidence does not aid decisionmaking, we do not present it.

Table 3. Criteria to rank strength of evidence

Grade	Definition
High	**High confidence that the evidence reflects the true effect.** Further research is very unlikely to change our confidence in the estimate of effect.
Moderate	**Moderate confidence that the evidence reflects the true effect.** Further research may change our confidence in the estimate of effect and may change the estimate.
Low	**Low confidence that the evidence reflects the true effect.** Further research is likely to change the confidence in the estimate of effect and is likely to change the estimate.
Insufficient	Evidence either is unavailable or does not permit a conclusion.

Assessing Applicability

We estimated applicability of the sample by evaluating the selection of children with migraine in observational studies and clinical trials.[68] Studies of community-dwelling children with 6 months or more followup with drug treatments had high applicability, as did large observational cohorts based on national registries, population-based effectiveness trials, and nationally representative administrative and clinical databases.

Peer Review and Public Commentary

We invited experts in migraine management fields and individuals representing stakeholder and user communities to provide external peer review of this report. AHRQ and an associate editor also provided comments. The draft report was posted on the AHRQ Web site for 4 weeks to elicit public comment. We addressed all reviewer comments and revised the text as appropriate. We documented all comments and our responses to them in a disposition of comments report that will be made available 3 months after the Agency posts the final review on the AHRQ Web site.

Results

Of 510 retrieved references, we excluded 104 at screening as not relevant to pediatric migraine, and we reviewed full texts of 312 references (Figure 2). We ultimately included 24 references of randomized controlled clinical trials, two abstracts of randomized controlled clinical trials, and 16 nonrandomized studies. We did not rank strength of evidence for two RCTs of flunarizine because, despite being commonly used elsewhere, this drug is not approved by the FDA. We found one eligible FDA review that evaluated a clinical trial of divalproex sodium used to prevent migraine headache in adolescents.[69]

Of 14 completed clinical trials registered in ClinicalTrials.gov, four were published. Publications occurred 1.8±1.2 years after study completion. Completion dates were missing for three completed unpublished studies of divalproex. Of the nine Phase III studies involving exclusively children, none posted the results on ClinicalTrials.gov. The results were not available for 4,001 subjects enrolled in studies involving children or 1,093 children enrolled in exclusive pediatric studies.

Appendix D provides evidence tables with the results from the included studies. Appendix E presents all excluded studies with exact reasons for exclusion.

Figure 2. Study flow*

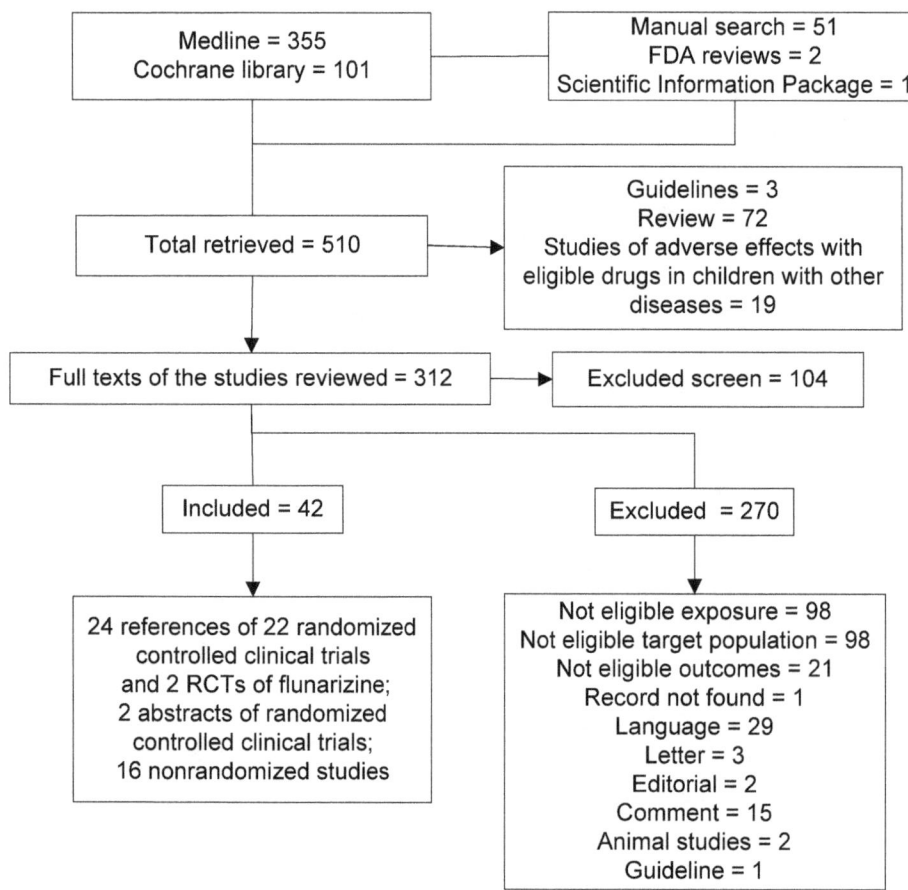

*References for RCTs included multiple publications and reanalyses of RCTs.

Study Overview

Characteristics

The results from the eligible studies were applicable to the target population. Most trials were conducted in Western countries and recruited children and adolescents in clinics. Only two trials recruited participants from the community. We analyzed baseline characteristics of the included children and concluded that enrolled patients represented the epidemiology of migraine in the target population (Table 4 and Appendix Table D1). Caucasian girls made up more than half of all enrolled subjects. Many enrolled subjects were overweight according to the mean age and mean body mass index. Children had migraine for an average 3.6 years, and suffered from an average of eight migraine attacks per month. Most trials defined migraine according to diagnostic criteria of the International Headache Society (Appendix Table D2). Reporting other characteristics of children was poor. More than half the trials failed to report family history of migraine, children's socioeconomic status, baseline comorbidity, prior treatments, overuse of drugs for acute migraine, or adherence to assigned treatments.

Based on infrequently reported trial flows, we estimated that investigators had to screen one to four children to enroll one (Appendix Table D3). Because we based our estimate on rarely reported study flow information in the original studies, it may have low applicability. The trials lasted an average of 20 weeks (ranging from 6 to 35 weeks) (Table 5). Attrition rates with active treatments averaged around 6.5 percent.

Risk of Bias

Of all included trials, we concluded low risk of bias in nine RCTs, medium risk of bias in six RCTs, and unclear risk of bias in five RCTs (Table 6). Most trials were double blind (Appendix Table D4); however, randomization was adequate in just 12 trials. Trials lasted an average of 20 weeks after a run-in period of 5.5 weeks (Appendix Table D1). We concluded high risk of bias in nonrandomized studies that did not address selection bias in study design and analyses.

Risk of bias differed depending on where the study was published. Some journals published RCTs with poorly reported trial design and conduct (Appendix Table D5). Most RCTs were published in the journal Headache; only half percent of all published RCTs in this journal had low risk of bias.

Risk of bias was associated with funding of the trials (Appendix Table D5). Industry-funded RCTs had lower risk of bias than trials funded by grants, combined, or other sources.

Trials enrolled in average 76 children (ranging from 14 to 305) and aimed to examine prevention of episodic migraine and adverse effects. Trials rarely reported statistical power to detect statistically significant differences in outcomes.

Key Question 1. What is the efficacy and comparative effectiveness of pharmacologic treatments for preventing migraine attacks in children?

Key Question 1a. How do preventive pharmacologic treatments affect patient-centered and intermediate outcomes when compared to placebo or no active treatment?

Efficacy RCTs examined migraine prevention with drugs versus placebo (Appendix Table D6).[70-88]

Half of the RCTs did not report ethical approval by institutional review boards or consent of the participants (Appendix Table D7). Most RCTs used a double-blind design (Appendix Table D8). Eligible trials defined clinically important migraine prevention as a complete cessation of migraine attacks and a reduction in monthly migraine frequency by ≥50 or 75 percent.

Off-Label Pharmacologic Agents

Table 7 summarizes the effectiveness of off-label pharmacologic agents for patient-centered outcomes. Here we present the effects of the drugs for both patient-centered and intermediate outcomes.

Antiepileptic Drugs

Topiramate

Topiramate, 50 to 200 mg/day, was no more effective than placebo in reducing monthly migraine attacks by ≥50 percent (two RCTs of 298 children, moderate-strength evidence) (Appendix Tables D9 and D10).[81,86] Topiramate, 100 mg/day, increased the likelihood of ≥50 percent reduction in migraine attacks in one of two RCTs that examined this association.[86] Topiramate increased the likelihood of ≥75 percent reduction in migraine days more often than placebo in a single double-blind RCT (Appendix Table D11).[81]

Using this statistically significant risk difference, we estimated that 181 children per 1,000 treated (95% CI, 52 to 311) would experience ≥75 percent reduction in migraine days due to topiramate, 200 mg/day.[81] Absolute reduction in migraine days with topiramate, 50 to 200 mg/day, was not better than with placebo in a pooled analysis of two double-blind RCTs (Appendix Table D12).

Divalproex

Divalproex sodium, 250 to 1,000 mg/day, was no more effective than placebo in reducing monthly migraine by ≥50 percent in one low-risk-of-bias RCT (305 children, low-strength evidence) (Appendix Table D13).[69,73]

Divalproex sodium in doses of 250, 500, or 1,000 mg/day was not better than placebo in reducing the number of migraine attacks, decreasing migraine days, or decreasing acute drug use (Appendix Tables D14-D16).[69,73]

Beta Blockers

Propranolol resulted in a complete cessation of migraine attacks more often than placebo (one RCT of 28 children, low-strength evidence) (Appendix Table D17).[79]

Two small RCTs examined the efficacy of propranolol. One small double-blind low-risk-of-bias RCT demonstrated that children experienced a complete cessation of migraine attacks more often with propranolol than with placebo (Appendix Table D18).[79] We estimated that 713 children per 1,000 treated would experience complete cessation of migraine with propranolol.[79] The same study separately examined reduction of migraine attacks by 50 percent and found no difference between propranolol and placebo.

In a second small crossover RCT, propranolol failed to show a significant reduction in migraine days compared with placebo (Appendix Table D19).[77]

Antidepressants

Compared with placebo, trazodone more effectively reduced the frequency and duration of migraine attacks by 1.6 per month and reduced duration of migraine attacks by 8.2 hours per attack (one RCT of 40 children, low-strength evidence).[70] A single small double-blind crossover RCT examined the efficacy of trazodone versus placebo (Appendix Table D20).[70] No studies examined reducing monthly migraine attacks by ≥50 percent or other patient-centered outcomes.

Calcium Channel Antagonists

Nimodipine was better than placebo in decreasing the number of migraine days (one RCT of 37 children, low-strength evidence). Nimodipine decreased the number of migraine days (mean difference 0.9, 95% CI, 0.5 to 1.3) (Appendix Table D21) but not the duration of migraine attacks.[76] No studies examined reducing monthly migraine attacks by ≥50 percent or other patient-centered outcomes.

Antiadrenergic Drugs

Clonidine was no more effective than placebo in reducing migraine duration or severity or reducing the use of drugs for acute treatment (one RCT of 57 children, low-strength evidence) (Appendix Table D22). The efficacy of the anti-adrenergic drug clonidine was examined in one small double-blind low-risk-of-bias RCT (Appendix Table D23).[71]

Magnesium Oxide

A single RCT demonstrated no significant differences with magnesium oxide and placebo in migraine frequency.[74] Magnesium oxide reduced severity of migraine attacks compared with placebo.[74] No studies examined reducing monthly migraine attacks by ≥50 percent or other patient-centered outcomes.

Key Question 1b. How do preventive pharmacologic treatments affect patient-centered and intermediate outcomes when compared to active pharmacologic treatments?

Limited evidence from individual RCTs suggested no differences in migraine prevention with examined drugs including propranolol, valproate, and topiramate.

Three RCTs examined comparative effectiveness of drugs for migraine prevention in children (Appendix Tables D24 and D25).[78,85,88] The trials had medium[78] or unclear risk of bias[85,88] (Appendix Table D26).

Two RCTs examined the comparative effectiveness of sodium valproate versus propranolol; the drugs did not differ significantly for achieving complete cessation of headache attacks or reduction by ≥50 percent from baseline frequency of migraine attacks (low-strength evidence) (Appendix Table D27).[78,88] Sodium valproate, 15 to 30 mg/kg/day, was more effective than propranolol, 2 to 3 mg/kg/day, in reducing baseline headache frequency by >70 percent in a single RCT (Appendix Table D28).[78] The drugs did not differ in effects for reducing migraine severity or use of acute drugs for migraine attacks.

One RCT of 48 children examined the comparative effectiveness of topiramate versus sodium valproate (low-strength evidence). The two drugs did not differ in their effects on migraine frequency, intensity, duration, or Pediatric Migraine Disability Assessment Score (Appendix Table D29).[85]

Key Question 1c. How do preventive pharmacologic treatments affect patient-centered and intermediate outcomes when compared to active nonpharmacologic treatments?

Limited evidence from individual RCTs suggested that the beta blockers propranolol and metoprolol were less effective than certain nonpharmacologic treatments, such as self-administered stress management and relaxation techniques, for preventing migraine in children. Two small RCTs compared drugs with active nonpharmacologic treatments (Appendix Tables D30 and D31).[75,77] We concluded unclear risk of bias in both trials because the authors provided insufficient details about methodology (Appendix Table D32).

One RCT examined comparative effectiveness of metoprolol versus a combined treatment involving stress management and either progressive relaxation training or stress management training that used specific relaxation exercises in response to usual migraine triggers such as an intrusively noisy radio program or specific tasks demanding cognitive effort. Stress management training also included objective measurements of changes in brain blood volume taken via photoplethysmograph. This RCT found no significant differences in the percentage of children who improved by ≥50 percent in the headache index (low-strength evidence) (Appendix Table D33).[75] In fact, metoprolol tended to be less effective in preventing migraine or reducing migraine severity than stress management combined with either progressive relaxation training or cephalic vasomotor feedback (Appendix Table D34).[75] The differences, however, did not achieve statistical significance.

One RCT (low-strength evidence) examined the comparative effectiveness of propranolol versus nonpharmacologic treatment (Appendix Table D35).[77] The trial found more frequent migraine with the drug than with self-hypnosis (mean difference of nine monthly migraine attacks, 95% CI, 4 to 14) (Appendix Table D35).[77]

Key Question 1d. How do preventive pharmacologic treatments combined with nondrug treatments affect patient-centered and intermediate outcomes when compared to pharmacologic treatments alone?

No studies compared combined pharmacologic and nondrug preventive treatments with monodrug therapy in children.

Key Question 1e1. How might dosing regimens or duration of treatments influence the effects of the treatments on patient-centered outcomes?

Four RCTs published in five articles[69,73,84,86,87] and one pooled analysis of three RCTs[82] examined the dose-response effects of preventive antiepileptic drugs in children (Appendix Tables D36 and D37). All RCTs were double blind with low risk of bias (Appendix Table D38).

Topiramate

The evidence did not support a dose-response association between increased doses of topiramate and reduction in migraine frequency or disability. A higher dose of topiramate compared to a lower dose (100 versus 25 mg) demonstrated no consistent significant difference in migraine prevention (Appendix Table D39).[84,86]

Higher doses of topiramate resulted in no greater reduction in disability score or migraine duration (Appendix Table D40).[84,86]

Divalproex Sodium

Higher doses of divalproex sodium (500 to 1,000 versus 250 mg/day) resulted in no significantly better migraine prevention in a single RCT that examined this association (Appendix Table D41). Higher doses of divalproex sodium resulted in no greater reduction in migraine days or acute drug use (Appendix Table D42).[69,73]

Key Question 1e2. How might approaches to drug management (such as patient care teams, integrated care, coordinated care, patient education, drug surveillance, or interactive drug monitoring) influence results?

Multidisciplinary migraine drug management, including cognitive-behavioral training, was more effective than a combination of usual care and education in preventing migraine in children and adolescents (one RCT of 68 children, low-strength evidence).[89]

A single RCT of 68 children and adolescents 10 to 18 years old examined internet-based multimodal drug management, including cognitive-behavioral training (CBT) or applied relaxation, compared to usual care (Appendix Table D43).[89]

The multimodal CBT intervention focused on stress management (perception of own stress symptoms, coping with stress), progressive relaxation techniques, cognitive restructuring (identification of dysfunctional cognitions regarding headache and self-assurance strategies such as being proactive and sensitive to one's own needs), and problem solving. The participants communicated through email with a multidisciplinary team of trial coordinators.[89] The applied relaxation included progressive relaxation, cue-controlled (triggered by key word or an image) relaxation, and differential relaxation.[89] Multimodal CBT was more effective than education in reducing migraine frequency by ≥50 percent (relative risk 4.0, 95% CI 1.0 to 16.0) (Appendix Table D44).[89] We estimated that 310 children per 1,000 treated with multimodal CBT would experience ≥50 percent reduction in migraine frequency (95% CI, 70 to 550). The effect, however, was not sustained at 6 months of followup.[89] Migraine frequency (Appendix Table D45) and quality of life did not differ with internet-based self-management versus an education program (Appendix Table D46).[89]

Key Question 2. What are the comparative harms from pharmacologic treatments for preventing migraine attacks in adults and children?

Key Question 2a. What are the harms from preventive pharmacologic treatments when compared to placebo or no active treatment?

Divalproex sodium resulted in treatment discontinuation due to adverse effects (Table 8). Topiramate significantly increased risk of weight loss, paresthesia, and upper respiratory tract infection.

Ten publications of randomized trials and one pooled analysis of three RCTs[82] examined the safety of drugs for migraine prevention in children (Appendix Table D47).[70-74,80-82,86,87] The trials included 1,046 children 12.6 years old with in average 10 monthly migraine attacks (Table 9). Half of the enrolled subjects were girls.

All RCTs were double blind (Table 10). Based on all risk of bias criteria, we concluded that six RCTs had low risk of bias and four RCTs had medium risk of bias.[74,80,81] Trials followed children for 19 weeks to assess harms (Table 11). Means of attrition rates were 10 percent with active treatments and 7 percent with control treatments.

Sixteen nonrandomized studies reported harms with migraine preventive drugs in children (Appendix Table D48).

Adverse Effects of Antiepileptic Drugs

Topiramate

Treatment discontinuation due to adverse effects was not greater with topiramate than placebo in a pooled analysis of two RCTs (low-strength evidence) (Table 12, Appendix Tables D49 and D50).[81,82,86,87]Nonrandomized studies suggested that 19 percent of children discontinued topiramate treatments due to bothersome adverse effects.[90]

A single RCT reported that 260 children per 1,000 treated with topiramate (95% CI, 30 to 480) experienced adverse effects (Appendix Table D51).[86] Our pooled analysis of individual adverse effects (Appendix Table D52) demonstrated a significant increase in risk of weight loss, paresthesia, and upper respiratory tract infection with topiramate. We estimated that of 1,000 treated with topiramate, 87 experienced unintended weight loss (95% CI, 24 to 150), and 105 were diagnosed with upper respiratory tract infection (95% CI, 29 to 182) (Table 13).[81,82,86]

Rates of the adverse effects did not differ between 50, 100, and 200 mg topiramate per day (Appendix Table D53). The results remain statistically nonsignificant from different statistical models (relative risk, absolute risk difference, arcsine transformed risk difference).

A single case report described development of the "Alice in Wonderland syndrome"[91] in which the treated girl described a distortion in her body image and a perception of disproportional body, arms, and head size. This event was associated with a dose of 75 mg/day of topiramate, but not with lower doses of the drug (Appendix Table D48).[91]

Divalproex Sodium

Treatment discontinuation due to adverse effects with divalproex sodium compared to placebo was greater with 1,000 mg/day but not with 250 mg/day in one RCTs (low-strength evidence) (Table 12).[69,73]

Treatment discontinuation due to treatment failure did not differ between divalproex sodium and placebo (Appendix Table D54).[73] A single RCT demonstrated that 80 children per 1,000 treated with divalproex sodium, 1,000 mg/day, would stop taking the drug due to intolerable adverse effects (95% CI, 9 to 151)[69,73] (Appendix Table D55).[69,73]

Nonrandomized studies suggested that 84 percent of children experienced adverse effects with divalproex,[92] and 17 percent discontinued treatment due to bothersome adverse effects.[93]

A single RCT examined risk of individual adverse effects and found no significant differences with divalproex versus placebo (Appendix Table D56).[73] This double-blind trial had low risk of bias but lacked power to detect significant differences in rare adverse events with the drug versus placebo (sparse data).[73] Upper respiratory tract infections were more common with larger doses of divalproex (Appendix Table D57).[73] The results differed depending on the statistical model used. Viral infections were more common with larger doses of divalproex in the models that obtained arcsine transformed risk difference (Appendix Table D57).[73]

Adverse Effects With Beta Blockers

A single RCT offered low-strength evidence that risk of any adverse effects did not differ between propranolol and placebo (Appendix Table D58).[80]

Adverse Effects With Antidepressants

A single low-risk-of-bias RCT offered low-strength evidence that treatment discontinuation for any reason did not differ between the antidepressant trazodone and placebo in 40 children with migraine (Appendix Table D59).[70] One retrospective chart review demonstrated that of 14 patients taking amitriptyline, 36 percent discontinued it at 16 weeks because of side effects.[94]

Adverse Effects With Antiadrenergic Drugs

Two RCTs reported treatment discontinuation due to adverse effects. One RCT demonstrated that risk of treatment discontinuation due to adverse effects did not differ between the anti-adrenergic drug clonidine and placebo (Table 12).[71] This double-blind RCT demonstrated that clonidine significantly increased risk of fatigue (Appendix Table D60).[71] We estimated that 220 children of 1,000 treated became fatigued (95% CI, 30 to 410) with clonidine.[71] Other adverse effects, including drowsiness or difficulty in reading, did not differ between clonidine and placebo.[72] A second small RCT failed to demonstrate any statistically significant increase in risk of adverse effects.[72]

Adverse Effects With Magnesium Oxide

A single RCT demonstrated no difference between magnesium oxide and placebo for risk of treatment discontinuation or for treatment discontinuation due to treatment failure or adverse effects (Appendix Table D61).[74]

Adverse Effects With Onabotulinumtoxin A

One small nonrandomized study demonstrated that 8 percent of adolescents treated with onabotulinumtoxin A 100U every 3 months experienced blurred vision and ptosis, and burning sensations at all injection sites[95] (Appendix Table D48).

Key Question 2b. What are the harms from preventive pharmacologic treatments when compared to active pharmacologic treatments?

Comparative Safety of Topiramate Versus Sodium Valproate

A single RCT (low-strength evidence) found no differences in any adverse effects with topiramate and sodium valproate administered for 12 weeks in 48 children with migraine (Appendix Table D62).[85]

Key Question 2c. How might approaches to drug management (such as patient care teams, integrated care, coordinated care, patient education, drug surveillance, or interactive drug monitoring) influence results?

We found no studies that examined how drug management can improve safety of migraine preventive medications in children.

Key Question 3. Which patient characteristics predict the effectiveness and safety of pharmacologic treatments for preventing migraine attacks in children and adults?

We found no studies that examined how specific characteristics of children could affect the effectiveness or safety of migraine preventive medications.

Table 4. Subject characteristics in randomized controlled clinical trials that examined migraine prevention in children

Drugs References for RCTs*	Age # RCTs / Mean [Min to Max]	% Female # RCTs / Mean [Min to Max]	Baseline Frequency of Migraine/Month # RCTs / Mean [Min to Max]	Duration of Migraine, Years # RCTs / Mean [Min to Max]	Obesity, BMI # RCTs / Mean [Min to Max]	Family History of Migraine, % # RCTs / Mean [Min to Max]
Topiramate[81-87]	7 / 12.6 [10.5 to 14.2]	7 / 56.9 [31.0 to 71.4]	5 / 9.6 [4.1 to 17.3]	1 / 4.2	2 / 23.3 [21.7 to 24.9]	0
Divalproex[69,73,96]	1 / 14.2	1 / 55.0	1 / 17.2	0	1 / 23.2	0
Valproate[69,73,96]	1 / 9.8	1 / 33.9	1 / 7.9	0	0	0
Propranolol[77-80]	2 / 9.5 [9.2 to 9.9]	4 / 40.6 [33.0 to 46.2]	3 / 10.3 [3.4 to 14.0]	1 / 4.0	0	3 / 66.8 [13.0 to 100.0]
Metoprolol[75]	1 / 11.3	1 / 39.5	1 / 5.4	1 / 4.7	0	0
Trazodone[70]	1 / 12.6	1 / 45.0	1 / 3.8	1 / 4.5	0	1 / 67.5
Nimodipine[76]	1 / 12.2	1 / 51.4	1 / 3.2	0	0	0
Clonidine[71,72]	1 / 11.0	2 / 41.4 [38.6 to 44.2]	1 / 3.5	0	0	1 / 90.7
Magnesium[74]	1 / 12.0	1 68.6	1 / 10.5	1 / 3.5	0	0
Drug management[89]	1 / 12.7	1 / 54.6	1 / 4.0	1 / 2.8	0	0
Total	17 / 11.8 [9.2 to 14.2]	20 / 49.9 [31.0 to 71.4]	16 / 8.4 [3.2 to 17.3]	6 / 3.6 [2.2 to 4.7]	3 / 23.3 [21.7 to 24.9]	5 / 75.0 [13.0 to 100.0]

BMI = body mass index; RCT = randomized controlled trial

*Include multiple publications of RCTs.

20

Table 5. Sample, duration, length of followup, and attrition in randomized controlled clinical trials that examined migraine prevention in children

Drug References for RCTs*	Duration of Run-In Period, Weeks # RCTs / Mean [Min to Max]	Total Sample Assigned to Treatment # RCTs / Mean [Min to Max]	Total Length of Followup, Weeks # RCTs / Mean [Min to Max]	Loss of Followup in Control Group, % # RCTs / Mean [Min to Max]	Loss of Followup in Active Group, % # RCTs / Mean [Min to Max]
Topiramate[81-87]	5 / 7.2 [4.0 to 9.0]	7 / 75.4 [14.0 to 162.0]	7 / 17.7 [12.0 to 26.0]	3 / 12.3 [4.0 to 24.7]	3 / 8.7 [4.5 to 11.4]
Divalproex[69,73,96]	1 / 6.0	1 / 305.0	1 / 12.0	1 / 5.5	1 / 3.9
Valproate[88]	0	1 / 120.0	1 / 12.0	0	0
Propranolol[77-80]	2 / 4.0 [4.0 to 4.0]	4 / 45.3 [32.0 to 63.0]	4 / 27.8 [24.0 to 35.0]	2 / 4.4 [3.3 to 5.5]	2 / 4.2 [3.3 to 5.1]
Metoprolol[75]	1 / 4.0	1 / 43.0	1 / 32.0	0	0
Trazodone[70]	1 / 4.0	1 / 40.0	1 / 28.0	0	0
Nimodipine[76]	0	1 / 37.0	1 / 28.0	0	0
Clonidine[71,72]	0	2 / 54.0 [51.0 to 57.0]	2 / 16.0 [8.0 to 24.0]	1 / 9.8	1 / 9.8
Magnesium[74]	1 / 4.0	1 / 118.0	1 / 16.0	0	0
Drug management[89]	0	1 / 68.0	1 / 6.0	0	
Total	11 / 5.5 [4.0 to 9.0]	20 / 75.73 [14.0 to 305.0]	20 / 19.9 [6.0 to 35.0]	7 / 8.7 [3.3 to 24.7]	7 / 6.5 [3.3 to 11.4]

RCT = randomized controlled trials

*include multiple publications of RCTs.

Table 6. Risk of bias in randomized controlled clinical trials that examined migraine prevention in children

Drugs References for RCTs*	Masking of the Treatment Status	Allocation Concealment	Adequacy of Randomization	Planned Intention To Treat Analysis	Risk of Bias	Total
Topiramate[81-87]	Double blind: 6 Open label: 1	Adequate: 2 Not adequate: 1 Unclear: 4	Adequate: 4 Not adequate: 3 Unclear: 0	Yes: 5 No: 0 Unclear: 2	Low: 4 Medium: 2 Unclear: 1	7
Divalproex[69,73,96]	Double blind: 1 Open label: 0	Adequate: 0 Not adequate: 0 Unclear: 1	Adequate: 1 Not adequate: 0 Unclear: 0	Yes: 1 No: 0 Unclear: 0	Low: 1 Medium: 0 Unclear: 0	1
Valproate[88]	Double blind: 0 Open label: 1	Adequate: 0 Not adequate: 0 Unclear: 1	Adequate: 1 Not adequate: 0 Unclear: 0	Yes: 0 No: 1 Unclear: 0	Low: 0 Medium: 0 Unclear: 1	1
Propranolol[77-80]	Double blind: 3 Open label: 1	Adequate: 0 Not adequate: 0 Unclear: 4	Adequate: 2 Not adequate: 1 Unclear: 1	Yes: 0 No: 1 Unclear: 3	Low: 1 Medium: 2 Unclear: 1	4
Metoprolol[75]	Double blind: 0 Open label: 1	Adequate: 0 Not adequate: 0 Unclear: 1	Adequate: 0 Not adequate: 1 Unclear: 0	Yes: 0 No: 0 Unclear: 1	Low: 0 Medium: 0 Unclear: 1	1
Trazodone[70]	Double blind: 1 Open label: 0	Adequate: 0 Not adequate: 0 Unclear: 1	Adequate: 0 Not adequate: 0 Unclear: 1	Yes: 0 No: 0 Unclear: 1	Low: 1 Medium: 0 Unclear: 0	1
Nimodipine[76]	Double blind: 1 Open label: 0	Adequate: 0 Not adequate: 0 Unclear: 1	Adequate: 1 Not adequate: 0 Unclear: 0	Yes: 0 No: 0 Unclear: 1	Low: 1 Medium: 0 Unclear: 0	1
Clonidine[71,72]	Double blind: 2 Open label: 0	Adequate: 0 Not adequate: 0 Unclear: 2	Adequate: 1 Not adequate: 0 Unclear: 1	Yes: 0 No: 1 Unclear: 1	Low: 1 Medium: 1 Unclear: 0	2
Magnesium[74]	Double blind: 1 Open label: 0	Adequate: 1 Not adequate: 0 Unclear: 0	Adequate: 0 Not adequate: 1 Unclear: 0	Yes: 1 No: 0 Unclear: 0	Low: 0 Medium: 1 Unclear: 0	1
Drug management[89]	Double blind: 0 Open label: 1	Adequate: 1 Not adequate: 0 Unclear: 0	Adequate: 0 Not adequate: 0 Unclear: 1	Yes: 1 No: 0 Unclear: 0	Low: 0 Medium: 0 Unclear: 1	1
Total	Double blind: 15 Open label: 5	Adequate: 4 Not adequate: 1 Unclear: 15	Adequate: 10 Not adequate: 6 Unclear: 4	Yes: 8 No: 2 Unclear: 10	Low: 9 Medium: 6 Unclear: 5	20

RCT = randomized controlled trial
*Include multiple publications of RCTs.

22

Table 7. Effects of preventive pharmacologic treatments on reduction in monthly migraine attacks

Outcome	Active	Control	RCTs Reference	Children	Rate Active, %	Rate Control, %	Relative Risk (95% CI)	Absolute Risk Difference (95% CI)	Number Needed To Treat (95% CI)	Attributable Events per 1,000 Treated (95% CI)	Strength of Evidence (Reason for Lowering)
Complete cessation of headache attacks	**Propranolol***	Placebo	1[79]	28	84.6	13.0	6.3 (1.7 to 23.5)	0.71 (0.45 to 0.97)	1 (1 to 2)	713 (452 to 974)	**Low** (imprecision in relative risk)
	Clonidine	Placebo	1[71]	57	10.7	24.1	0.4 (0.1 to 1.5)	-0.13 (-0.33 to 0.06)	NS	NS	Low (imprecision)
	Sodium valproate	Propranolol	2[78,88]	183	17.1	15.4	1.2 (0.6 to 2.2)	0.02 (-0.09 to 0.12)	NS	NS	Low (medium risk of bias, imprecision)
Reduction by ≥50% in migraine attack frequency	Topiramate	Placebo	2[81,86]	298	58.2	45.7	1.3 (0.9 to 1.8)	0.15 (-0.06 to 0.37)	NS	NS	Moderate (medium risk of bias)
Reduction by ≥50% in migraine attack frequency	Divalproex sodium	Placebo	1[73]	305	49.0	45.0	1.1 (0.8 to 1.5)	0.04 (-0.12 to 0.20)	NS	NS	Low (imprecision)
Reduction by ≥75% in migraine attack frequency	Propranolol	Placebo	1[79]	28	7.7	0.0	3.4 (0.2 to 77.6)	0.08 (-0.11 to 0.26)	NS	NS	Low (imprecision)
1-2 migraine frequency/month	Clonidine	Placebo	1[71]	57	32.1	27.6	1.2 (0.5 to 2.6)	0.05 (-0.19 to 0.28)	NS	NS	Low (imprecision)
Reduction by ≥50% in migraine attack frequency	Sodium valproate	Propranolol	2[88]	183	69.5	74.3	0.9 (0.7 to 1.2)	-0.07 (-0.30 to 0.15)	NS	NS	Low (medium risk of bias, imprecision)

23

Table 7. Effects of preventive pharmacologic treatments on reduction in monthly migraine attacks (continued)

Outcome	Active	Control	RCTs Reference	Children	Rate Active, %	Rate Control, %	Relative Risk (95% CI)	Absolute Risk Difference (95% CI)	Number Needed To Treat (95% CI)	Attributable Events per 1,000 Treated (95% CI)	Strength of Evidence (Reason for Lowering)
Reduction by ≥50% in the headache index**	**Metoprolol***	**Progressive relaxation training + stress management**	1[75]	28	**38.5**	80.0	0.5 (0.2 to 1.0)	**-0.42 (-0.75 to -0.08)**	**-2 (-12 to -1)**	**-415 (-748 to -82)**	**Low** (unclear risk of bias, imprecision)
	Metoprolol	Cephalic vasomotor feedback + stress management	1[75]	28	38.5	53.3	0.7 (0.3 to 1.7)	-0.15 (-0.51 to 0.22)	NS	NS	Low (unclear risk of bias, imprecision)
Reduction for need for temporary drug therapy for single attacks	Clonidine	Placebo	1[71]	57	50.0	34.5	1.5 (0.8 to 2.7)	0.16 (-0.10 to 0.41)	NS	NS	Low (imprecision)
Improvement in Pediatric Migraine Disability Assessment Score	Topiramate	Sodium valproate	1[85]	48	NA	NA	Mean difference -0.9 (-5.6 to 3.8)		NS	NS	Low (unclear risk of bias, imprecision)

CI = confidence interval; NA = not applicable; NS = not significant (number needed to treat and number of attributable events were calculated for statistically significant differences); RCT = randomized controlled trial

*Bold = significant differences at 95% confidence level when 95% CI of attributable events does not include 0.

**Intensity of headache episodes.

24

Table 8. Evidence of treatment discontinuation due to adverse effects with migraine preventive drugs versus placebo in children

Drug	RCTs Reference	Children	Conclusion	Strength of evidence
Divalproex sodium, 1,000 mg	1[69,73]	148	Divalproex sodium 1,000 mg resulted in greater treatment discontinuation rates vs. placebo	Low (imprecision)
Topiramate, 50-200 mg	2[81,86,87]	298	Topiramate 50-200 mg, did not result in greater treatment discontinuation rates vs. placebo	Low (imprecision, medium risk of bias)
Clonidine	1[71]	57	Clonidine 25-50 μg did not result in greater rates of treatment discontinuation vs. placebo; the data is sparse	Insufficient
Magnesium	1[74]	118	Magnesium did not result in greater rates of treatment discontinuation vs. placebo	Low (medium risk of bias, imprecision)

Table 9. Subject characteristics in randomized controlled clinical trials that examined harms with interventions for migraine prevention in children

Drugs References for RCTs*	Age # RCTs / Mean [Min to Max]	% Females # RCTs / Mean [Min to Max]	Baseline Frequency of Migraine/Month # RCTs / Mean [Min to Max]	Duration of Migraine, Years # RCTs / Mean [Min to Max]	Obesity, BMI # RCTs / Mean [Min to Max]	Family History of Migraine, % # RCTs / Mean [Min to Max]
Topiramate[81,82,86,87]	4 / 13.4 [11.1 to 14.2]	4 / 60.4 [48.4 to 71.0]	2 / 4.7 [4.1 to 5.2]	0	2 / 23.3 [21.7 to 24.9]	0
Divalproex[69,73,96]	1 / 14.2	1 / 55.0	1 / 17.2	0	1 / 23.2	0
Propranolol[80]	0	1 / 46.2	1 / 14.0	0	0	1 / 13.0
Trazodone[70]	1 / 12.6	1 / 45.0	1 / 3.8	1 / 4.5	0	1 / 67.5
Clonidine[71,72]	1 / 11.0	2 / 41.4 [38.6 to 44.2]	1 / 3.5]	0	0	1 / 90.7
Magnesium[74]	1 / 12.0	1 / 68.6	1 / 10.5	1 / 3.5	0	0
Total	8 / 12.6 [11.0 to 14.2]	10 / 49.9 [38.6 to 71.0]	7 / 10.1 [3.5 to 17.2]	2 / 4.0 [3.5 to 4.5]	3 / 23.3 [21.7 to 24.9]	3 / 57.1 [13.0 to 67.5]

BMI = body mass index; RCT = randomized controlled trial
*Includes multiple publications of RCTs.

25

Table 10. Risk of bias in randomized controlled clinical trials that examined harms with interventions for migraine prevention in children

Drugs References for RCTs*	Masking of the Treatment Status	Allocation Concealment	Adequacy of Randomization	Planned Intention To Treat Analysis	Risk of Bias	Total
Topiramate[81,82,86,87]	Double blind: 4 Open label: 0	Adequate: 2 Not adequate: 0 Unclear: 2	Adequate: 2 Not adequate: 2 Unclear: 0	Yes: 4 No: ITT: 0 Unclear: 0	Low: 3 Medium: 1 Unclear: 0	4
Divalproex[69,73,96]	Double blind: 1 Open label: 0	Adequate: 0 Not adequate: 0 Unclear: 1	Adequate: 1 Not adequate: 0 Unclear: 0	Yes: 1 No: ITT: 0 Unclear: 0	Low: 1 Medium: 0 Unclear: 0	1
Propranolol[80]	Double blind: 1 Open label: 0	Adequate: 0 Not adequate: 0 Unclear: 1	Adequate: 0 Not adequate: 1 Unclear: 0	Yes: 0 No: ITT: 0 Unclear: 1	Low: 0 Medium: 1 Unclear: 0	1
Trazodone[70]	Double blind: 1 Open label: 0	Adequate: 0 Not adequate: 0 Unclear: 1	Adequate: 0 Not adequate: 0 Unclear: 1	Yes: 0 No: ITT: 0 Unclear: 1	Low: 1 Medium: 0 Unclear: 0	1
Clonidine[71,72]	Double blind: 2 Open label: 0	Adequate: 0 Not adequate: 0 Unclear: 2	Adequate: 1 Not adequate: 0 Unclear: 1	Yes: 0 No: ITT: 1 Unclear: 1	Low: 1 Medium: 1 Unclear: 0	2
Magnesium[74]	Double blind: 1 Open label: 0	Adequate: 1 Not adequate: 0 Unclear: 0	Adequate: 0 Not adequate: 1 Unclear: 0	Yes: 1 No: ITT: 0 Unclear: 0	Low: 0 Medium: 1 Unclear: 0	1
Total	Double blind: 10 Open label: 0	Adequate: 3 Not adequate: 0 Unclear: 7	Adequate: 4 Not adequate: 4 Unclear: 2	Yes: 6 No: ITT: 1 Unclear: 3	Low: 6 Medium: 4 Unclear: 0	10

ITT = intention to treat; RCT = randomized controlled trial
*Includes multiple publications of RCTs.

26

Table 11. Sample, duration, length of followup, and attrition in randomized controlled clinical trials that examined harms with interventions for migraine prevention in children

Drugs References for RCTs*	Duration of Run-In Period, Weeks # RCTs / Mean [Min to Max]	Total Sample Assigned to Treatment # RCTs / Mean [Min to Max]	Total Length of Followup, Weeks # RCTs / Mean [Min to Max]	Loss of Followup Control Group, % # RCTs / Mean [Min to Max]	Loss of Followup in Active Group, % # RCTs / Mean [Min to Max]
Topiramate[81,82,86,87]	4 / 8.0 [6.0 to 9.0]	4 / 105.5 [51.0 to 162.0]	4 / 21.0 [16.0 to 26.0]	3 / 12.3 [4.0 to 24.7]	3 / 8.7 [4.5 to 11.4]
Divalproex[69,73,96]	1 / 6.0	1 / 305.0	1 / 12.0	1 / 5.5	1 / 3.9
Propranolol[80]	1 / 4.0	1 / 53.0	1 / 26.0	1 / 3.3	1 / 3.3
Trazodone[70]	1 / 4.0	1 / 40.0	1 / 28.0	0	0
Clonidine[71,72]	0	2 / 54.0 [51.0 to 57.0]	2 / 16.0 [8.0 to 24.0]	1 / 9.8	1 / 9.8
Magnesium[74]	1 / 4.0	1 / 118.0	1 / 16.0	0	0
Total	8 / 6.3 [4.0 to 9.0]	10 / 103.9 [40.0 to 305.0]	10 / 18.8 [8.0 to 28.0]	6 / 9.5 [3.3 to 24.7]	6 / 6.6 [3.3 to 11.4]

RCT = randomized controlled trial
*Includes multiple publications of RCTs.

Table 12. Treatment discontinuation due to adverse effects with migraine preventive drugs versus placebo in children

Drug	RCTs References*	Children	Rate With Drug, %	Rate With Placebo, %	Relative Risk (95% CI)	Absolute Risk Difference (95% CI)	Number Needed To Treat (95% CI)	Attributable Events per 1,000 Treated (95% CI)	Strength of Evidence (Reason for Lowering)
Divalproex sodium, 1,000 mg**	**1[69,73]**	**148**	**9.3**	**1.4**	**6.8 (0.9 to 54)**	**0.08 (0.01 to 0.16)**	**13 (7 to 111)**	**80 (9 to 151)**	**Low** (imprecision)
Topiramate, 50-100 mg	2[81,86,87]	298	7	3.5	2.1 (0.7 to 6.3)	0.04 (-0.02 to 0.1)	NS	NS	Low (imprecision, medium risk of bias)
Clonidine	1[71]	57	3.5	0	3.1 (0.1 to 73.1)	0.04 (-0.06 to 0.13)	NS	NS	Insufficient
Magnesium	1[74]	118	5.2	1.7	3.1 (0.3 to 29.0)	0.04 (-0.03 to 0.10)	NS	NS	Low (medium risk of bias, imprecision)

CI = confidence interval; NS = not significant (number needed to treat and number of attributable events were calculated for statistically significant differences)
*Includes multiple publications of RCTs.
**Bold = significant differences at 95% confidence level when 95% CI of absolute risk difference do not include 0. The entire line is bold.

27

Table 13. Adverse effects with antiepileptic drugs for migraine prevention in children

Adverse Effect	Drug	References for RCTs*	Children in Analyses	Rate With Drug, %	Rate With Placebo, %	Relative Risk (95% CI)	Absolute Risk Difference (95% CI)	Number Needed To Treat To Harm (95% CI)	Attributable Events per 1,000 Treated (95% CI)
Any adverse event**	**Divalproex sodium**	1[73,97]	305	66.6	57.8	1.2 (1.0 to 1.3)	0.09 (0.01 to 0.18)	11 (5 to 200)	94 (5 to 183)
Abdominal pain	Topiramate	3[81,82,86]	373	10.4	9.9	1.0 (0.6 to 1.9)	0.00 (-0.06 to 0.06)	NS	NS
Anorexia	Topiramate	3[81,82,86,87]	373	11.8	5.9	1.8 (0.9 to 3.8)	0.05 (0.00 to 0.11)	NS	NS
Dizziness	Topiramate	2[82,86,87]	531	4.6	5.9	0.7 (0.1 to 3.7)	-0.03 (-0.14 to 0.08)	NS	NS
Fatigue	Topiramate	3[81,82,86,87]	373	6.8	8.6	0.8 (0.4 to 1.6)	-0.02 (-0.08 to 0.04)	NS	NS
Injury	Topiramate	3[81,82,86]	373	8.1	8.6	0.9 (0.5 to 1.8)	0.00 (-0.06 to 0.06)	NS	NS
Nausea	Topiramate	2[81,86]	298	6.0	6.0	1.0 (0.4 to 2.6)	0.00 (-0.06 to 0.06)	NS	NS
Paresthesia**	**Topiramate**	3[81,82,86]	373	**14.5**	**5.3**	**2.6 (1.2 to 5.6)**	**0.09 (0.05 to 0.14)**	**11 (7 to 22)**	**92 (45 to 140)**
Sinusitis	Topiramate	3[81,82,86]	373	8.1	5.3	1.2 (0.5 to 2.5)	0.02 (-0.03 to 0.07)	NS	NS
Somnolence	Topiramate	3[81,82,86,87]	305	8.1	5.0	1.4 (0.6 to 3.6)	0.03 (-0.02 to 0.09)	NS	NS
Treatment discontinuation	Topiramate	3[81,82,86,87]	490	19.6	25.8	0.8 (0.5 to 1.2)	-0.03 (-0.11 to 0.05)	NS	NS
Upper respiratory tract infection**	**Topiramate**	3[81,82,86]	373	21.7	11.2	**1.8 (1.1 to 3.1)**	**0.11 (0.03 to 0.18)**	**10 (5 to 34)**	**105 (29 to 182)**
Weight decrease**	**Topiramate**	3[81,82,86]	373	20.8	12.5	**2.0 (1.2 to 3.2)**	**0.09 (0.02 to 0.15)**	**11 (7 to 42)**	**87 (24 to 150)**

CI = confidence interval; NS = not significant (number needed to treat and number of attributable events were calculated for statistically significant differences); RCT = randomized controlled trial

*Includes multiple publications which contributed to meta-analyses only once.

**Bold = significant differences at 95% confidence level when 95% CI of absolute risk difference do not include 0.

28

Discussion

Our comprehensive review identified limited evidence about benefits and harms with migraine preventive drugs in children. Migraine prevention in children was examined in 24 publications of 22 RCTs that enrolled 1,578 children. Only one drug, the beta blocker propranolol, prevented migraine more effectively than placebo (Table 14). Propranolol (60 to 120 mg/day) would result in complete cessation of migraine attacks in 713 per 1,000 treated children (95% CI, 452 to 974) (low-strength evidence from a single RCT).[79] Topiramate, divalproex, clonidine, trazodone, and magnesium oxide failed to prevent migraine in children. Divalproex sodium, 1000 mg/day, resulted in greater rates of treatment discontinuation due to adverse effects (Table 12). Topiramate significantly increased risk of weight loss, paresthesia, and upper respiratory tract infection (Table 13).

No studies examined whether specific characteristics of children modify the effectiveness or safety of preventive drugs. Treatment effects may differ between children and adolescents. Published trials did not provide treatment effects among age subgroups.

Clinical decisions about drugs and nonpharmacologic treatment for migraine prevention in children should include a careful estimation of the balance of benefits and harms. Our review confirmed previously published conclusions about the efficacy of propranolol for migraine prevention in children.[98] However, nonpharmacologic treatments demonstrated better benefit-to-harm ratios than drugs in head-to-head RCTs.[75,77,99] Individualized multimodal drug management showed promising results.[89] Other complex disease management interventions including school-based psychological interventions and drug management programs have both demonstrated positive results in treating acute headache attacks, but neither has been examined for migraine prevention.[100,101] RCTs have not yet examined other drug management interventions, including integrated care, coordinated care, patient education, drug surveillance, and interactive drug monitoring.

The off-label antiepileptic drugs, clonidine and trazodone failed to demonstrate efficacy for migraine prevention but resulted in bothersome adverse effects. Previously published reviews reported bothersome adverse effects with antiepileptic drugs in children with migraine[102,103] or epilepsy.[104] Off-label use of the antidepressant trazodone in children with migraine was not effective. We could not conclude the effectiveness of other antidepressants for preventing migraine in children, nor could we determine whether adverse effects of antidepressants are similar when used for children with migraine compared to children with depression. We do know that antidepressants may increase risk of suicidal behavior in children and adolescents.[105] Use of off-label psychotropic drugs for migraine prevention could be justified in children with psychiatric comorbidity;[106] however, trials available for review did not report presence of comorbid illnesses in enrolled patients.

In fact, few available trials examined the seriousness or bothersomeness of harms with drugs. Clinicians considering off-label drugs for children with migraine have very limited evidence about balance between benefits and harms for informed decisionmaking. Few clinical trials followed the recommendations from the Task Force on Adverse Events in Migraine Trials of the International Headache Society[107] when testing safety of the drugs in children. Future fully powered trials involving children with migraine should examine long-term safety with preventive drugs, regardless of the investigators' perceptions about the causal association between the drugs and the detected harms.

Table 14. Evidence of migraine prevention in children

Outcome	Active	Control	RCTs Reference	Conclusion	Strength of Evidence (Reason for Lowering)
Complete cessation of headache attacks	Propranolol	Placebo	1[79]	Propranolol was better than placebo in achieving complete cessation of migraine attacks.	Low (imprecision)
	Clonidine	Placebo	1[71]	Clonidine was not better than placebo in achieving complete cessation of migraine attacks.	Low (imprecision)
	Sodium valproate	Propranolol	2[78,88]	Sodium valproate and propranolol had no significant differences in complete cessation of headache attacks.	Low (medium risk of bias imprecision)
Reduction by 50% in migraine attack frequency	Topiramate	Placebo	2[81,86]	Topiramate, 50-200 mg/d, did not increase rate of reduction in migraine by ≥50%.	Moderate (medium risk of bias)
Reduction by ≥50% in migraine attack frequency	Divalproex sodium	Placebo	1[73]	Divalproex sodium, 250-1,000 mg/d did not increase rate of reduction in migraine by 50%.	Low (imprecision)
1-2 migraine frequency/month	Clonidine	Placebo	1[71]	Clonidine did not increase rate of reduction in migraine.	Low (imprecision)
Reduction by ≥50% in migraine attack frequency	Sodium valproate	Propranolol	2[78,88]	Sodium valproate and propranolol had no significant differences in reduction of migraine attack by ≥50% from baseline with both drugs.	Low (medium risk of bias, imprecision)
	Metoprolol	Progressive relaxation training + stress management	1[75]	Metoprolol was less effective in reduction by ≥50% in Headache Index.	Low (unclear risk of bias, imprecision)
Reduction by ≥50% in migraine attack frequency	Metoprolol	Cephalic vasomotor feedback + stress management	1[75]	Metoprolol and cephalic vasomotor feedback + stress management had no significant differences in reduction by ≥50% in Headache Index.	Low (unclear risk of bias, imprecision)
Reduction for need for temporary drug therapy for single attacks	Clonidine	Placebo	1[71]	Clonidine did not decrease drug utilization for acute migraine attacks.	Low (imprecision)
Improvement in Pediatric Migraine Disability Assessment Score	Topiramate	Sodium valproate	1[85]	Topiramate and sodium valproate had no significant differences in Pediatric Migraine Disability Assessment Score.	Low (unclear risk of bias, imprecision)

RCT = randomized controlled trial

30

Strength of evidence of drug benefits and harms was low in most cases due to risk of bias and imprecise estimates from underpowered RCTs. Reporting quality of trials was poor with few trials providing detailed information about prior or concomitant treatments, comorbidities, family history, socioeconomic status, drug overuse, and other important characteristics of children. On average, the trials lasted 20 weeks, and therefore did not provide sufficiently long-term evidence for benefits and harms with drugs that could be recommended for preventive use over very long time periods. The optimal duration of preventive treatment and sustained benefits and harms with preventive drugs in children with migraine remain unclear.[28,108]

Our review has limitations. We did not conclude strength of evidence for flunarizine, which has been reported to be effective in preventing migraines in children, because this drug has not been approved by the FDA. One low-risk-of-bias Italian RCT suggested that flunarizine resulted in ≥50 percent reduction in migraine attacks in 500 children per 1,000 treated (95% CI, 260 to 740).[109] We do not know why flunarizine was never approved in the United States. We requested the FDA review of this drug and received a response that stated: "Any information on an application if submitted by a firm to the FDA that did not yet receive approval, belongs to the manufacturer/sponsor developing the drug (21 CFR 314.430)." We did not contact the sponsors directly to inquire about products under development. Comprehensive review of nonpharmacologic treatments was beyond our scope.

Our comprehensive literature search in several databases, trial registries, and the FDA reviews detected a very low publication rate of registered completed clinical trials involving children. We do not know why the studies were not published. We assume publication bias but did not contact the investigators of completed trials for unpublished data. We requested additional data from the sponsors of completed trials but received few responses. Thus, we know neither the results from unpublished trials nor how many unregistered studies have been conducted and never published. We relied on reported information and did not contact study authors for additional details about the trials, including design, execution, or poorly reported results that we could not reproduce.

Key Messages

- Propranolol was more effective than placebo for preventing migraine in children, with no bothersome adverse effects that could lead to treatment discontinuation.
- Antiepileptics were no more effective than placebo in preventing migraine but resulted in increased risk of adverse effects.
- Internet-based self-management with multimodal CBT was better than education in preventing migraine in children and adolescents at 6 weeks but not at 6 months of followup.
- Reporting quality of studies involving children is poor.

Our report offers insights for future research on preventive treatments for childhood migraine, all of which should be conducted according to the recently published Standards for Research in Child Health group (Table 15).[110-115] Future randomized trials should examine the comparative effectiveness of multimodal drug and disease management; long-term benefits, safety, and adherence with preventive treatments; and the role of specific characteristics of children that could modify benefits and harms with preventive drugs.

Table 15. Future research needs

Key Question	Results of Literature Review	Types of Studies Needed To Answer Question	Future Research Recommendation

What is the efficacy and comparative effectiveness of pharmacologic treatments for preventing migraine attacks in children?	Only one drug, beta blocker propranolol prevented migraine more effectively than placebo in a single RCT. Multidisciplinary drug management including cognitive-behavioral training was more effective than usual care with educational intervention in preventing migraine in children and adolescents.	Randomized trials; analyses of administrative databases to examine practice patterns of off label drug use and comparative effectiveness on health care utilization	Analyze efficacy of drugs that were effective for migraine prevention in children and adults:
			a. Beta blockers including
			  - Propranolol
			  - Timolol
			  - Metoprolol
			  - Atenolol
			  - Nadolol
			  - Bisoprolol
			  - Nebivolol
			b. ACE inhibitors lisinopril and captopril
			c. Angiotensin II Antagonists including
			  - Candesartan
			  - Telmisartan
			Analyze efficacy and comparative effectiveness of multidisciplinary community, family, or school based migraine drug management interventions.
			Analyze administrative databases (Medicaid, health insurance databases) to examine preventive drug utilization and effectiveness of preventive drugs on emergency room utilization.
			Trials should examine long-term treatment effectiveness based on patient centered outcomes including complete cessation of migraine attack or reduction in monthly migraine attacks by ≥50%; quality of life; migraine related disability; success with schooling.

What are the comparative harms from pharmacologic treatments for preventing migraine attacks in children?	Divalproex sodium, 1000 mg/day) resulted in treatment discontinuation due to adverse effects.	Randomized trials; analysis of administrative databases
		Case-series and case reports about harms with preventive drugs
		Creation of the registry with adverse effects form preventive drugs in children with migraine
			Analyze long-term safety of drugs with good benefits/harms profile in adults:
			a. Beta blockers
			b. ACE inhibitors lisinopril and captopril
			c. Angiotensin II Antagonists including
			  - Candesartan
			  - Telmisartan
			Analyze administrative databases (Medicaid, health insurance databases) to examine preventive drug utilization and comparative safety of preventive drugs on diagnosed adverse effects that lead to treatment discontinuation or additional health care utilization (emergency room visits, hospitalization).

Table 15. Future research needs (continued)

Key Question	Results of Literature Review	Types of Studies Needed To Answer Question	Future Research Recommendation
Which characteristics of children predict the effectiveness and safety of pharmacologic treatments for preventing migraine attacks?	No studies examined how children's' characteristics can improve effectiveness or safety of migraine preventive medications in children.	Randomized trials; analysis of administrative databases	Examine with interaction models how children age, sex, race, ethnicity, puberty, socioeconomic status, family history, comorbid psychiatric and other diseases can modify benefits and harms with preventive drugs. Examine benefits and harms with preventive drugs in subgroups by children age, sex, race, ethnicity, puberty, socioeconomic status, family history, comorbid psychiatric and other diseases. Examine effectiveness and safety of preventive drugs and multidisciplinary interventions in children with chronic migraine, migraine with vs. without aura, and those for whom previous preventive treatments failed.

33

Future studies should also specifically examine the effects and risks of off-label drug use for migraine prevention in children. Randomized trials have examined only a few pharmacologic agents, but practicing clinicians use many off-label drugs to treat children, and little is known about the comparative effectiveness or safely of the drug classes used. Large observational studies, including the American Migraine Prevalence and Prevention study, relied on self-reported use of preventive medications and did not assess exact drug use or effectiveness.[1] The few available studies of off-label drug use in children show that 5 percent of all antiepileptic drug prescriptions were for migraine.[116] The National Ambulatory Medical Care Surveys from 2001 to 2004 demonstrated that 62 percent of outpatient pediatric visits included off-label prescribing; 86 percent of those prescriptions were for pain.[117] European studies demonstrated that about 30 percent of hospitalized children[118] and 40 percent of children in outpatient settings received off-label drug prescriptions.[119] European observational studies found a significantly higher risk of adverse effects with off-label drugs, concluding an improper balance of benefits and risks with off-label drugs in pediatric patients.[119,120]

As a first step, the comparative effectiveness and safety of off-label drugs used for migraine prevention in children should be examined by analyzing administrative databases. Such analyses could, for example, shed light on practice patterns in migraine prevention and provide insight into the comparative effectiveness of preventive drugs for reducing visits to emergency rooms. Based on these analyses, RCTs could be designed to examine the drugs that demonstrate the most favorable ratios of benefits to harms. Future studies should also assess the efficacy and comparative effectiveness of multidisciplinary migraine drug management interventions based in the community, family, or school.

Trials should examine treatment effectiveness based on patient-centered outcomes, including complete cessation of migraine attack or reduction in monthly migraine attacks by ≥ 50 percent, quality of life, migraine-related disability, and success with schooling. Studies should examine subgroups of children identified by age, sex, race, ethnicity, puberty, socioeconomic status, family history, and comorbid psychiatric conditions and other diseases. Studies should also examine the effectiveness and safety of preventive drugs and multidisciplinary interventions in children with chronic migraine, migraine with versus without aura, and those for whom previous preventive treatments have failed.

Existing clinical research policy does not guarantee availability of the results from all studies involving children. Results are unavailable for more than half of the studies involving children, revealing a substantial publication bias.[121] Registration and posting of results on ClinicalTrials.gov should be mandatory for all studies involving children.[121]

References

1. Diamond S, Bigal ME, Silberstein S, et al. Patterns of diagnosis and acute and preventive treatment for migraine in the United States: results from the American Migraine Prevalence and Prevention study. Headache. 2007 Mar;47(3):355-63. PMID 17371352.

2. Lipton RB, Scher AI, Kolodner K, et al. Migraine in the United States: epidemiology and patterns of health care use. Neurology. 2002 Mar 26;58(6):885-94. PMID 11914403.

3. Bigal ME, Lipton RB, Winner P, et al. Migraine in adolescents: association with socioeconomic status and family history. Neurology. 2007 Jul 3;69(1):16-25. PMID 17606878.

4. Hernandez-Latorre MA, Roig M. Natural history of migraine in childhood. Cephalalgia. 2000 Jul;20(6):573-9. PMID 11075841.

5. Lewis DW. Pediatric migraine. Neurol Clin. 2009 May;27(2):481-501. PMID 19289227.

6. Goadsby PJ, Raskin NH. Chapter 15. Headache. In: Fauci AS, Braunwald E, Kasper DL, Hauser SL, Longo DL, Jameson JL, et al., eds. Harrison's principles of internal medicine. 17th ed. New York: The McGraw-Hill Companies; 2008.

7. Headache Classification Subcommittee of the International Headache Society. The International Classification of Headache Disorders: 2nd edition. Cephalalgia. 2004;24 Suppl 1:9-160. PMID 14979299.

8. Silberstein SD. Preventive migraine treatment. Neurol Clin. 2009 May;27(2):429-43. PMID 19289224.

9. Lipton RB, Manack A, Ricci JA, et al. Prevalence and burden of chronic migraine in adolescents: results of the chronic daily headache in adolescents study (C-dAS). Headache. 2011 May;51(5):693-706. PMID 21521206.

10. Bille B. A 40-year follow-up of school children with migraine. Cephalalgia. 1997 Jun;17(4):488-91; discussion 7. PMID 9209767.

11. Guidetti V, Galli F. Evolution of headache in childhood and adolescence: an 8-year follow-up. Cephalalgia. 1998 Sep;18(7):449-54. PMID 9793696.

12. Lipton RB, Stewart WF, Diamond S, et al. Prevalence and burden of migraine in the United States: data from the American Migraine Study II. Headache. 2001 Jul-Aug;41(7):646-57. PMID 11554952.

13. Damen L, Bruijn JK, Verhagen AP, et al. Symptomatic treatment of migraine in children: a systematic review of medication trials. Pediatrics. 2005 Aug;116(2):e295-302. PMID 16061583.

14. Sprenger T, Goadsby PJ. Migraine pathogenesis and state of pharmacological treatment options. BMC Medicine. 2009;7:71. PMID 19917094.

15. Sanchez-Del-Rio M, Reuter U, Moskowitz MA. New insights into migraine pathophysiology. Curr Opin Neurol. 2006 Jun;19(3):294-8. PMID 16702838.

16. Rapoport AM. Acute and prophylactic treatments for migraine: present and future. Neurol Sci. 2008 May;29 Suppl 1:S110-22. PMID 18545911.

17. Stafford RS. Regulating off-label drug use--rethinking the role of the FDA. N Engl J Med. 2008 Apr 3;358(14):1427-9. PMID 18385495.

18. Fraguas D, Merchan-Naranjo J, Laita P, et al. Metabolic and hormonal side effects in children and adolescents treated with second-generation antipsychotics. Journal of Clinical Psychiatry. 2008 Jul;69(7):1166-75. PMID 18588363.

19. Correll CU, Carlson HE. Endocrine and metabolic adverse effects of psychotropic medications in children and adolescents. J Am Acad Child Adolesc Psychiatry. 2006 Jul;45(7):771-91. PMID 16832314.

20. Pappagallo M, Silva R. The effect of atypical antipsychotic agents on prolactin levels in children and adolescents. J Child Adolesc Psychopharmacol. 2004 Fall;14(3):359-71. PMID 15650493.

21. Kumra S, Oberstar JV, Sikich L, et al. Efficacy and tolerability of second-generation antipsychotics in children and adolescents with schizophrenia. Schizophr Bull. 2008 Jan;34(1):60-71. PMID 17923452.

22. Dubois D. Toxicology and overdose of atypical antipsychotic medications in children: does newer necessarily mean safer? Curr Opin Pediatr. 2005 Apr;17(2):227-33. PMID 15800418.

23. Silberstein S, Tfelt-Hansen P, Dodick DW, et al. Guidelines for controlled trials of prophylactic treatment of chronic migraine in adults. Cephalalgia. 2008 May;28(5):484-95. PMID 18294250.

24. Schroeder BM. AAFP/ACP-ASIM release guidelines on the management and prevention of migraines. Am Fam Physician. 2003 Mar 15;67(6):1392, 5-7. PMID 12674472.

25. Olesen J, Bousser MG, Diener HC, et al. New appendix criteria open for a broader concept of chronic migraine. Cephalalgia. 2006 Jun;26(6):742-6. PMID 16686915.

26. Lewis D, Ashwal S, Hershey A, et al. Practice parameter: pharmacological treatment of migraine headache in children and adolescents: report of the American Academy of Neurology Quality Standards Subcommittee and the Practice Committee of the Child Neurology Society. Neurology. 2004 Dec 28;63(12):2215-24. PMID 15623677.

27. Gunner KB, Smith HD, Ferguson LE. Practice guideline for diagnosis and management of migraine headaches in children and adolescents: Part two. J Pediatr Health Care. 2008 Jan-Feb;22(1):52-9. PMID 18174091.

28. Geraud G, Lanteri-Minet M, Lucas C, et al. French guidelines for the diagnosis and management of migraine in adults and children. Clin Ther. 2004 Aug;26(8):1305-18. PMID 15476911.

29. Evers S, Afra J, Frese A, et al. EFNS guideline on the drug treatment of migraine--revised report of an EFNS task force. Eur J Neurol. 2009 Sep;16(9):968-81. PMID 19708964.

30. Dowson AJ, Lipscombe S, Sender J, et al. New guidelines for the management of migraine in primary care. Curr Med Res Opin. 2002;18(7):414-39. PMID 12487508.

31. Morey SS. Guidelines on migraine: part 4. General principles of preventive therapy. Am Fam Physician. 2000 2000 Nov 15;62(10):2359-60. PMID 11126860.

32. Silberstein SD. Practice parameter: evidence-based guidelines for migraine headache (an evidence-based review): report of the Quality Standards Subcommittee of the American Academy of Neurology. Neurology. 2000 Sep 26;55(6):754-62. PMID 10993991.

33. Schuurmans A, van Weel C. Pharmacologic treatment of migraine. Comparison of guidelines. Can Fam Physician. 2005 Jun;51:838-43. PMID 15986940.

34. Solomon S. New appendix criteria open for a broader concept of chronic migraine (Comment on: Cephalagia 2006 Jun:26(6):742-6). Cephalalgia. 2007 May;27(5):469; author reply -70. PMID 17448186.

35. U.S. Food and Drug Administration. FDA News Release: FDA Approves Botox to Treat Chronic Migraine. 2010. http://www.fda.gov/NewsEvents/Newsroom/PressAnnouncements/ucm229782.htm. Accessed on July 25 2012.

36. Whitlock EP, Lopez SA, Chang S, et al. AHRQ series paper 3: identifying, selecting, and refining topics for comparative effectiveness systematic reviews: AHRQ and the effective health-care program. J Clin Epidemiol. 2010 May;63(5):491-501. PMID 19540721.

37. Slutsky J, Atkins D, Chang S, et al. AHRQ series paper 1: comparing medical interventions: AHRQ and the Effective Health-Care Program. J Clin Epidemiol. 2010 May;63(5):481-3. PMID 18834715.

38. Helfand M, Balshem H. AHRQ series paper 2: principles for developing guidance: AHRQ and the Effective Health-Care Program. J Clin Epidemiol. 2010 May;63(5):484-90. PMID 19716268.

39. Liberati A, Altman DG, Tetzlaff J, et al. The PRISMA statement for reporting systematic reviews and meta-analyses of studies that evaluate health care interventions: explanation and elaboration. Annals of Internal Medicine. 2009 Aug 18;151(4):W65-94. PMID 19622512.

40. White CM, Ip S, McPheeters ML, et al. Chapter 11. Using existing systematic reviews to replace de novo processes in conducting comparative effectiveness reviews. Methods Guide for Effectiveness and Comparative Reviews. AHRQ Publication No. 10(11)-EHC063-EF. Rockville, MD: Agency for Healthcare Resarch and Quality: March 2011; 2009:136-51. Available at www.effectivehealthcare.ahrq.gov.

41. Harris RP, Helfand M, Woolf SH, et al. Current methods of the US Preventive Services Task Force: a review of the process. Am J Prev Med. 2001 Apr;20(3 Suppl):21-35. PMID 11306229.

42. Rothner AD. Complicated migraine and migraine variants. Curr Pain Headache Rep. 2002 Jun;6(3):233-9. PMID 12003695.

43. Hansen JM, Thomsen LL, Olesen J, et al. Calcitonin gene-related peptide does not cause the familial hemiplegic migraine phenotype. Neurology. 2008 Sep 9;71(11):841-7. PMID 18779512.

44. Norris S, Atkins D, Bruening W, et al. Chapter 4. Selecting observational studies for comparing medical interventions. Methods Guide for Effectiveness and Comparative Reviews. AHRQ Publication No. 10(11)-EHC063-EF. Rockville, MD: Agency for Healthcare Research and Quality. March 2011:56-68. Available at: www.effectivehealthcare.ahrq.gov.

45. Higgins J, Green S, eds. Cochrane handbook for systematic reviews of interventions. Version 5.1.0. London: The Cochrane Collaboration; 2011.

46. Chou R, Aronson N, Atkins D, et al. AHRQ series paper 4: assessing harms when comparing medical interventions: AHRQ and the Effective Health-Care Program. J Clin Epidemiol. 2008 Sep 25;63(5):502-12. PMID 18823754.

47. Higgins JP, Altman DG, Gotzsche PC, et al. The Cochrane Collaboration's tool for assessing risk of bias in randomised trials. BMJ. 2011;343:d5928. PMID 22008217.

48. Viswanathan M, Berkman ND. Development of the RTI Item Bank on Risk of Bias and Precision of Observational Studies AHRQ Methods for Effective Health Care. 2011 Sep Studies;Rockville (MD): Agency for Healthcare Research and Quality (US)(Report No.: 11-EHC028-EF)PMID 22191112.

49. van der Velde G, van Tulder M, Cote P, et al. The sensitivity of review results to methods used to appraise and incorporate trial quality into data synthesis. Spine (Phila Pa 1976). 2007 Apr 1;32(7):796-806. PMID 17414916.

50. Herbison P, Hay-Smith J, Gillespie WJ. Adjustment of meta-analyses on the basis of quality scores should be abandoned. J Clin Epidemiol. 2006 Dec;59(12):1249-56. PMID 17098567.

51. Wallace BC, Schmid CH, Lau J, et al. Meta-Analyst: software for meta-analysis of binary, continuous and diagnostic data. BMC Med Res Methodol. 2009;9:80. PMID 19961608.

52. Egger M, Smith GD, Altman DG. Systematic reviews in health care: meta-analysis in context. 2nd ed. London: BMJ Books; 2001.

53. Fu R, Gartlehner G, Grant M, et al. Chapter 9. Conducting quantitative synthesis when comparing medical interventions. Methods Guide for Effectiveness and Comparative Effectiveness Reviews. AHRQ Publication No. 10(11)-EHC063-EF. Rockville, MD: Agency for Healthcare Research and Quality. March 2011:104-19. Available at: http://effectivehealthcare.ahrq.gov.

54. Rucker G, Schwarzer G, Carpenter J, et al. Why add anything to nothing? The arcsine difference as a measure of treatment effect in meta-analysis with zero cells. Stat Med. 2009 Feb 28;28(5):721-38. PMID 19072749.

55. Bradburn MJ, Deeks JJ, Berlin JA, et al. Much ado about nothing: a comparison of the performance of meta-analytical methods with rare events. Stat Med. 2007 Jan 15;26(1):53-77. PMID 16596572.

56. Sweeting MJ, Sutton AJ, Lambert PC. What to add to nothing? Use and avoidance of continuity corrections in meta-analysis of sparse data. Stat Med. 2004 May 15;23(9):1351-75. PMID 15116347.

57. Stijnen T, Hamza TH, Ozdemir P. Random effects meta-analysis of event outcome in the framework of the generalized linear mixed model with applications in sparse data. Stat Med. 2010 Dec 20;29(29):3046-67. PMID 20827667.

58. Friedrich JO, Adhikari NK, Beyene J. Ratio of means for analyzing continuous outcomes in meta-analysis performed as well as mean difference methods. Journal of Clinical Epidemiology. 2011 May;64(5):556-64. PMID 21447428.

59. Owens DK, Lohr KN, Atkins D, et al. AHRQ series paper 5: grading the strength of a body of evidence when comparing medical interventions-Agency for Healthcare Research and Quality and the Effective Health-Care Program. J Clin Epidemiol. 2010 May;63(5):513-23. PMID 19595577.

60. Viechtbauer W. Confidence intervals for the amount of heterogeneity in meta-analysis. Stat Med. 2007 Jan 15;26(1):37-52. PMID 16463355.

61. Knapp G, Biggerstaff BJ, Hartung J. Assessing the amount of heterogeneity in random-effects meta-analysis. Biom J. 2006 Apr;48(2):271-85. PMID 16708778.

62. DerSimonian R, Laird N. Meta-analysis in clinical trials. Control Clin Trials. 1986 Sep;7(3):177-88. PMID 3802833.

63. Ebrahim S. The use of numbers needed to treat derived from systematic reviews and meta-analysis. Caveats and pitfalls. Eval Health Prof. 2001 Jun;24(2):152-64. PMID 11523384.

64. Altman DG. Confidence intervals for the number needed to treat. BMJ. 1998 Nov 7;317(7168):1309-12. PMID 9804726.

65. Guyatt G, Oxman AD, Kunz R, et al. GRADE guidelines 6. Rating the quality of evidence-imprecision. J Clin Epidemiol. 2011 Aug 10PMID 21839614.

66. Sterne JA, Sutton AJ, Ioannidis JP, et al. Recommendations for examining and interpreting funnel plot asymmetry in meta-analyses of randomised controlled trials. BMJ. 2011;343:d4002. PMID 21784880.

67. Guyatt GH, Oxman AD, Santesso N, et al. GRADE guidelines 12. Preparing Summary of Findings tables-binary outcomes. J Clin Epidemiol. 2012 May 18PMID 22609141.

68. Aschengrau A, Seage GR. Essentials of epidemiology in public health. Sudbury, MA: Jones and Bartlett; 2003.

69. U.S. Food and Drug Administration. Clinical Review of Divalproex Sodium. 2008.

70. Battistella PA, Ruffilli R, Cernetti R, et al. A placebo-controlled crossover trial using trazodone in pediatric migraine. Headache. 1993 Jan;33(1):36-9. PMID 8436497.

71. Sillanpää M. Clonidine prophylaxis of childhood migraine and other vascular headache. A double blind study of 57 children. Headache; 1977. p. 28-31.

72. Sills M, Congdon P, Forsythe I. Clonidine and childhood migraine: a pilot and double-blind study. Dev Med Child Neurol. 1982 Dec;24(6):837-41. PMID 6218003.

73. Apostol G, Cady RK, Laforet GA, et al. Divalproex extended-release in adolescent migraine prophylaxis: results of a randomized, double-blind, placebo-controlled study. Headache. 2008 Jul;48(7):1012-25. PMID 18705027.

74. Wang F, Van Den Eeden SK, Ackerson LM, et al. Oral magnesium oxide prophylaxis of frequent migrainous headache in children: a randomized, double-blind, placebo-controlled trial. Headache. 2003 Jun;43(6):601-10. PMID 12786918.

75. Sartory G, Muller B, Metsch J, et al. A comparison of psychological and pharmacological treatment of pediatric migraine. Behav Res Ther. 1998 Dec;36(12):1155-70. PMID 9745800.

76. Battistella PA, Ruffilli R, Moro R, et al. A placebo-controlled crossover trial of nimodipine in pediatric migraine. Headache. 1990 Apr;30(5):264-8. PMID 2191938.

77. Olness K, MacDonald JT, Uden DL. Comparison of self-hypnosis and propranolol in the treatment of juvenile classic migraine. Pediatrics. 1987 Apr;79(4):593-7. PMID 3822681.

78. Bidabadi E, Mashouf M. A randomized trial of propranolol versus sodium valproate for the prophylaxis of migraine in pediatric patients. Paediatric Drugs. 2010 Aug 1;12(4):269-75. PMID 20593910.

79. Ludvigsson J. Propranolol used in prophylaxis of migraine in children. Acta neurologica Scandinavica; 1974. p. 109-15.

80. Forsythe WI, Gillies D, Sills MA. Propanolol ('Inderal') in the treatment of childhood migraine. Developmental medicine and child neurology; 1984. p. 737-41.

81. Winner P, Pearlman EM, Linder SL, et al. Topiramate for migraine prevention in children: a randomized, double-blind, placebo-controlled trial. Headache. 2005 Nov-Dec;45(10):1304-12. PMID 16324162.

82. Winner P, Gendolla A, Stayer C, et al. Topiramate for migraine prevention in adolescents: a pooled analysis of efficacy and safety. Headache. 2006 Nov-Dec;46(10):1503-10. PMID 17115983.

83. Lakshmi CV, Singhi P, Malhi P, et al. Topiramate in the prophylaxis of pediatric migraine: a double-blind placebo-controlled trial. J Child Neurol. 2007 Jul;22(7):829-35. PMID 17715274.

84. Lewis D, Paradiso E. A double-blind, dose comparison study of topiramate for prophylaxis of basilar-type migraine in children: a pilot study. Headache. 2007 Nov-Dec;47(10):1409-17. PMID 18052950.

85. Unalp A, Uran N, Ozturk A. Comparison of the effectiveness of topiramate and sodium valproate in pediatric migraine. J Child Neurol. 2008 Dec;23(12):1377-81. PMID 19073842.

86. Lewis D, Winner P, Saper J, et al. Randomized, double-blind, placebo-controlled study to evaluate the efficacy and safety of topiramate for migraine prevention in pediatric subjects 12 to 17 years of age. Pediatrics. 2009 Mar;123(3):924-34. PMID 19255022.

87. Pandina GJ, Ness S, Polverejan E, et al. Cognitive effects of topiramate in migraine patients aged 12 through 17 years. Pediatr Neurol. 2010 Mar;42(3):187-95. PMID 20159428.

88. Ashrafi MR, Shabanian R, Zamani GR, et al. Sodium Valproate versus Propranolol in paediatric migraine prophylaxis. Eur J Paediatr Neurol. 2005;9(5):333-8. PMID 16120482.

89. Trautmann E, Kroner-Herwig B. A randomized controlled trial of Internet-based self-help training for recurrent headache in childhood and adolescence. Behav Res Ther. 2010 Jan;48(1):28-37. PMID 19782343.

90. Cruz MJ, Valencia I, Legido A, et al. Efficacy and tolerability of topiramate in pediatric migraine. Pediatric Neurology. 2009 Sep;41(3):167-70. PMID 19664530.

91. Jurgens TP, Ihle K, Stork JH, et al. "Alice in Wonderland syndrome" associated with topiramate for migraine prevention. J Neurol Neurosurg Psychiatry. 2011 Feb;82(2):228-9. PMID 20571045.

92. Apostol G, Lewis DW, Laforet GA, et al. Divalproex sodium extended-release for the prophylaxis of migraine headache in adolescents: results of a stand-alone, long-term open-label safety study. Headache. 2009 Jan;49(1):45-53. PMID 19040679.

93. Pakalnis A, Greenberg G, Drake ME, Jr., et al. Pediatric migraine prophylaxis with divalproex. Journal of Child Neurology. 2001 Oct;16(10):731-4. PMID 11669346.

94. Sorge F, Barone P, Steardo L. Amitriptyline as a prophylactic for migraine in children. Acta Neurologica. 1982;4(5):362-7.

95. Chan VW, McCabe EJ, MacGregor DL. Botox treatment for migraine and chronic daily headache in adolescents. Journal of Neuroscience Nursing. 2009 Oct;41(5):235-43. PMID 19835236.

96. Apostol G, Pakalnis A, Laforet GA, et al. Safety and tolerability of divalproex sodium extended-release in the prophylaxis of migraine headaches: results of an open-label extension trial in adolescents. Headache. 2009 Jan;49(1):36-44. PMID 19040678.

97. Sorge F, De Simone R, Marano E, et al. Flunarizine in prophylaxis of childhood migraine. A double-blind, placebo-controlled, crossover study. Cephalalgia; 1988. p. 1-6.

98. Victor S, Ryan SW. Drugs for preventing migraine headaches in children. Cochrane Database of Systematic Reviews. 2003(4):CD002761. PMID 14583952.

99. Damen L, Bruijn J, Koes BW, et al. Prophylactic treatment of migraine in children. Part 1. A systematic review of non-pharmacological trials. Cephalalgia. 2006 Apr;26(4):373-83. PMID 16556238.

100. Larsson B, Carlsson J, Fichtel A, et al. Relaxation treatment of adolescent headache sufferers: results from a school-based replication series. Headache. 2005 Jun;45(6):692-704. PMID 15953302.

101. Fichtel A, Larsson B. Relaxation treatment administered by school nurses to adolescents with recurrent headaches. Headache. 2004 Jun;44(6):545-54. PMID 15186298.

102. Jayapal S, Maheshwari N. Question 3. Topiramate for chronic migraine in children. Arch Dis Child. 2011 Mar;96(3):318-21. PMID 21317129.

103. Damen L, Bruijn J, Verhagen AP, et al. Prophylactic treatment of migraine in children. Part 2. A systematic review of pharmacological trials. Cephalalgia. 2006 May;26(5):497-505. PMID 16674757.

104. Connock M, Frew E, Evans BW, et al. The clinical effectiveness and cost-effectiveness of newer drugs for children with epilepsy. A systematic review. Health Technol Assess. 2006 Mar;10(7):iii, ix-118. PMID 16545206.

105. Bridge JA, Iyengar S, Salary CB, et al. Clinical response and risk for reported suicidal ideation and suicide attempts in pediatric antidepressant treatment: a meta-analysis of randomized controlled trials. JAMA. 2007 Apr 18;297(15):1683-96. PMID 17440145.

106. Breslau N. Psychiatric comorbidity in migraine. Cephalalgia. 1998 Aug;18 Suppl 22:56-8; discussion 8-61. PMID 9793713.

107. Tfelt-Hansen P, Bjarnason NH, Dahl, et al. Evaluation and registration of adverse events in clinical drug trials in migraine. Cephalalgia. 2008 Jul;28(7):683-8. PMID 18498392.

108. Wasiewski WW. Preventive therapy in pediatric migraine. Journal of Child Neurology. 2001 Feb;16(2):71-8. PMID 11292228.

109. Sorge F, Marano E. Flunarizine v. placebo in childhood migraine. A double-blind study. Cephalalgia. 1985 May;5 Suppl 2:145-8. PMID 2861907.

110. Sinha IP, Altman DG, Beresford MW, et al. Standard 5: Selection, Measurement, and Reporting of Outcomes in Clinical Trials in Children. Pediatrics. 2012 June 1, 2012;129(Supplement 3):S146-S52.

111. van der Tweel I, Askie L, Vandermeer B, et al. Standard 4: Determining Adequate Sample Sizes. Pediatrics. 2012 June 1, 2012;129(Supplement 3):S138-S45.

112. Ellenberg S, Fernandes RM, Saloojee H, et al. Standard 3: Data Monitoring Committees. Pediatrics. 2012 June 1, 2012;129(Supplement 3):S132-S7.

113. Hartling L, Hamm M, Klassen T, et al. Standard 2: Containing Risk of Bias. Pediatrics. 2012 June 1, 2012;129(Supplement 3):S124-S31.

114. Caldwell PHY, Dans L, de Vries MC, et al. Standard 1: Consent and Recruitment. Pediatrics. 2012 June 1, 2012;129(Supplement 3):S118-S23.

115. Hartling L, Wittmeier KDM, Caldwell P, et al. StaR Child Health: Developing Evidence-Based Guidance for the Design, Conduct, and Reporting of Pediatric Trials. Pediatrics. 2012 June 1, 2012;129(Supplement 3):S112-S7.

116. van de Vrie-Hoekstra NW, de Vries TW, van den Berg PB, et al. Antiepileptic drug utilization in children from 1997-2005--a study from the Netherlands. Eur J Clin Pharmacol. 2008 Oct;64(10):1013-20. PMID 18618103.

117. Bazzano AT, Mangione-Smith R, Schonlau M, et al. Off-label prescribing to children in the United States outpatient setting. Acad Pediatr. 2009 Mar-Apr;9(2):81-8. PMID 19329098.

118. Choonara I, Conroy S. Unlicensed and off-label drug use in children: implications for safety. Drug Safety. 2002;25(1):1-5. PMID 11820908.

119. Horen B, Montastruc JL, Lapeyre-Mestre M. Adverse drug reactions and off-label drug use in paediatric outpatients. Br J Clin Pharmacol. 2002 Dec;54(6):665-70. PMID 12492616.

120. Ufer M, Kimland E, Bergman U. Adverse drug reactions and off-label prescribing for paediatric outpatients: a one-year survey of spontaneous reports in Sweden. Pharmacoepidemiol Drug Saf. 2004 Mar;13(3):147-52. PMID 15072113.

121. Shamliyan T, Kane RL. Clinical research involving children: registration, completeness, and publication. Pediatrics. 2012 May;129(5):e1291-300. PMID 22529271.

Abbreviations

AHRQ	Agency for Healthcare Research and Quality
ARD	Absolute risk difference
CBT	Cognitive behavioral training
CI	Confidence interval
EPC	Evidence-based Practice Center
FDA	Food and Drug Administration
ICHD-II	International Classification of Headache Disorders (second edition)
KQ	Key questions
MeSH	Medical Subject Heading
PICOTS	Population, Intervention, Comparator, Outcome, Timing, and Setting
PRISMA	Preferred Reporting Items for Systematic Review and Meta-Analysis
RCT	Randomized controlled trial
TEP	Technical Expert Panel

Appendix A. Literature Search

January 2011
PubMed

#	Strings	N
#8	Search "Migraine Disorders"[Mesh] AND "Migraine Disorders"[Mesh] Limits: Humans, Meta-Analysis, English	97
#7	Search "Migraine Disorders"[Mesh] AND "Migraine Disorders"[Mesh] Limits: Humans, Randomized Controlled Trial, English	907

#	Strings	N
#71	Search migraine NOT acute Limits: Humans, Randomized Controlled Trial, English	655
#70	Search migraine Limits: Humans, Randomized Controlled Trial, English	1040
#66	Search melatonin AND migraine	55
#67	Search melatonin AND migraine Limits: Humans, Clinical Trial, Randomized Controlled Trial, English	7
#64	Search "Brain-Derived Neurotrophic Factor"[Mesh] AND migraine	6
#63	Search "Brain-Derived Neurotrophic Factor"[Mesh] AND migraine Limits: Humans, Clinical Trial, Randomized Controlled Trial, English	1
#62	Search "Brain-Derived Neurotrophic Factor"[Mesh] Limits: Humans, Clinical Trial, Randomized Controlled Trial, English	94
#58	Search Risperidone AND migraine Limits: Humans, Clinical Trial, Randomized Controlled Trial, English	0
#57	Search Paliperidone AND migraine Limits: Humans, Clinical Trial, Randomized Controlled Trial, English	0
#56	Search Methiothepin AND migraine Limits: Humans, Clinical Trial, Randomized Controlled Trial, English	0
#55	Search Metergoline AND migraine Limits: Humans, Clinical Trial, Randomized Controlled Trial, English	0
#53	Search Lisuride AND migraine Limits: Humans, Clinical Trial, Randomized Controlled Trial, English	5
#51	Search Bromocriptine AND migraine Limits: Humans, Clinical Trial, Randomized Controlled Trial, English	4
#50	Search Zotepine AND migraine Limits: Humans, Clinical Trial, Randomized Controlled Trial, English	0
#49	Search Ziprasidone AND migraine Limits: Humans, Clinical Trial, Randomized Controlled Trial, English	0
#48	Search Trifluoperazine AND migraine Limits: Humans, Clinical Trial, Randomized Controlled Trial, English	0
#47	Search Tenilapine AND migraine Limits: Humans, Clinical Trial, Randomized Controlled Trial, English	0
#46	Search Sulpiride AND migraine Limits: Humans, Clinical Trial, Randomized Controlled Trial, English	1
#45	Search Spiperone AND migraine Limits: Humans, Clinical Trial, Randomized Controlled Trial, English	0
#44	Search Sertindole AND migraine Limits: Humans, Clinical Trial, Randomized Controlled Trial, English	0
#43	Search Olanzapine AND migraine Limits: Humans, Clinical Trial, Randomized Controlled Trial, English	0
#42	Search Loxapine AND migraine Limits: Humans, Clinical Trial, Randomized Controlled Trial, English	0
#41	Search Ketanserin AND migraine Limits: Humans, Clinical Trial, Randomized Controlled Trial, English	0
#40	Search Imipramine AND migraine Limits: Humans, Clinical Trial, Randomized Controlled Trial, English	0
#39	Search Fluperlapine AND migraine Limits: Humans, Clinical Trial, Randomized Controlled Trial, English	0

#38	Search **Fluphenazine AND migraine** Limits: Humans, Clinical Trial, Randomized Controlled Trial, English	0
#36	Search **Cyproheptadine AND migraine** Limits: Humans, Clinical Trial, Randomized Controlled Trial, English	9
#35	Search **Clozapine AND migraine** Limits: Humans, Clinical Trial, Randomized Controlled Trial, English	0
#33	Search **Clomipramine AND migraine** Limits: Humans, Clinical Trial, Randomized Controlled Trial, English	2
#32	Search **Aripiprazole AND migraine** Limits: Humans, Clinical Trial, Randomized Controlled Trial, English	0
#31	Search **Amoxapine AND migraine** Limits: Humans, Clinical Trial, Randomized Controlled Trial, English	0
#29	Search **Amitriptyline AND migraine** Limits: Humans, Clinical Trial, Randomized Controlled Trial, English	34
#28	Search **Amitriptyline AND migraine** Limits: Humans, English	150
#27	Search **5-HT7 AND migraine** Limits: Humans, English	12
#24	Search **5-HT7** Limits: Humans, English	150
#13	Search **Quetiapine AND migraine** Limits: Humans, English	5
#21	Search **"Antipsychotic Agents "[Pharmacological Action] AND migraine** Limits: Humans, Clinical Trial, Randomized Controlled Trial, English	41
#20	Search **"Antipsychotic Agents "[Pharmacological Action] AND migraine** Limits: Humans, English	206
#19	Search **"Antipsychotic Agents "[Pharmacological Action]** Limits: Humans, English	51308
#11	Search **5-HT2A AND migraine** Limits: Humans, English	14
#10	Search **5-HT2A antagonists AND migraine** Limits: Humans, English	3
#7	Search **5-HT2A antagonists** Limits: Humans, English	394
#5	Search **Alpha-2 agonists AND migraine** Limits: Humans, English	6
#4	Search **Alpha-2 agonists AND migraine**	17

#84	Search **telcagepant AND migraine** Limits: Humans, Clinical Trial, Randomized Controlled Trial, English	4
#83	Search **olcegepant AND migraine** Limits: Humans, Clinical Trial, Randomized Controlled Trial, English	0
#82	Search **Arachidonic cascade modulators** Limits: Humans, Clinical Trial, Randomized Controlled Trial, English	0
#80	Search **tonabersat) AND migraine** Limits: Humans, Clinical Trial, Randomized Controlled Trial, English	6
#79	Search **dextromethorphan AND migraine** Limits: Humans, Clinical Trial, Randomized Controlled Trial, English	0
#78	Search **dextromethorphan AND migraine NOT acute** Limits: Humans, Clinical Trial, Randomized Controlled Trial, English	0
#77	Search **loxapine AND migraine NOT acute** Limits: Humans, Clinical Trial, Randomized Controlled Trial, English	0
#76	Search **prochlorperazine AND migraine NOT acute** Limits: Humans, Clinical Trial, Randomized Controlled Trial, English	8
#75	Search **prochlorperazine AND migraine** Limits: Humans, Clinical Trial, Randomized Controlled Trial, English	20

August, 2011

#	Strings	N
#15	Search **Phenelzine AND migraine** Limits: Humans, Journal Article, English	11
#14	Search **Bupropion AND migraine** Limits: Humans, Journal Article, English	1
#13	Search **Imipramine AND migraine** Limits: Humans, Journal Article, English	15
#12	Search **Imipramine AND headache** Limits: Humans, Journal Article, English	60
#11	Search **Doxepin AND headache** Limits: Humans, Journal Article, English	15
#9	Search **Desipramine AND headache** Limits: Humans, Journal Article, English	13
#10	Search **Desipramine AND migraine** Limits: Humans, Journal Article, English	1
#7	Search **Protriptyline AND headache** Limits: Humans, Journal Article, English	4
#6	Search **Protriptyline AND migraine** Limits: Humans, Journal Article, English	0

Updated search in Ovid; 1948 to November Week 3 2011

#	Searches	Results
1	exp migraine disorders/dt	5944
2	exp migraine disorders/pc	1669
3	ad.fs.	998247
4	2 and 3	286
5	1 or 4	6112
6	1 or 2	7065
7	exp "off-label use"/	519
8	off label.mp.	2412
9	7 or 8	2412
10	6 and 9	14
11	exp calcium channel blockers/	68976
12	exp antihypertensive agents/	216956
13	exp antidepressive agents/	113058
14	exp anticonvulsants/	111349
15	exp botulinum toxin type a/	4832
16	exp alzheimer disease/dt	8107
17	11 or 12 or 13 or 14 or 15 or 16	476372
18	6 and 17	1675
19	5 or 10 or 18	6489
20	limit 19 to (humans and yr="2000 -Current")	3195
21	limit 20 to updaterange="mesz(20111121020154-20111121091315]"	0

Search for systematic reviews:

Searches	Results
Search systematic[sb] AND (quetiapine) AND child	16
Search systematic[sb] AND (Telmisartan) AND child	1
Search systematic[sb] AND (Captopril) AND child	5
Search systematic[sb] AND (Enalapril) AND child	2
Search systematic[sb] AND (Femoxetine) AND child	0
Search systematic[sb] AND (Metoprolol) AND child	4
Search systematic[sb] AND (acebutolol) AND child	0
Search systematic[sb] AND (bisoprolol) AND child	0
Search systematic[sb] AND (Atenolol) AND child	2
Search systematic[sb] AND (opipramol) AND child	0
Search systematic[sb] AND (Nadolol) AND child	0
Search systematic[sb] AND (Oxprenolol) AND child	0
Search systematic[sb] AND (Alprenolol) AND child	0
Search systematic[sb] AND (Labetalol) AND child	1
Search systematic[sb] AND (Timolol) AND child	2
Search systematic[sb] AND (Propranolol) AND child	17
Search systematic[sb] AND (Pindolol) AND child	0
Search systematic[sb] AND (Pindolol)	18
Search systematic[sb] AND (Rizatriptan) AND child	6
Search systematic[sb] AND (Zolmitriptan) AND child	5
Search systematic[sb] AND (Frovatriptan) AND child	0
Search systematic[sb] AND (Almotriptan) AND child	1
Search systematic[sb] AND (Sumatriptan) AND child	13
Search systematic[sb] AND (Venlafaxine) AND child	8
Search systematic[sb] AND (Paroxetine) AND child	13
Search systematic[sb] AND (citalopram) AND child	12
Search systematic[sb] AND (fluvoxamine) AND child	12
Search systematic[sb] AND (Nicardipine) AND child	1
Search systematic[sb] AND (Verapamil) AND child	4
Search systematic[sb] AND (Nimodipine) AND child	5
Search systematic[sb] AND (Nifedipine) AND child	4
Search systematic[sb] AND (Telcagepant) AND child	0

Search	Results
Search systematic[sb] AND (Olanzapine) AND child	18
Search systematic[sb] AND (aripiprazole) AND child	16
Search systematic[sb] AND (Pizotifen) AND child	9
Search systematic[sb] AND (Lasmiditan) AND child	0
Search systematic[sb] AND (Lasmiditan hydrochloride) AND child	0
Search systematic[sb] AND (Quinazoline) AND child	4
Search systematic[sb] AND (Piperazine) AND child	1
Search systematic[sb] AND (Clonidine) AND child	28
Search systematic[sb] AND (nortriptyline) AND child	4
Search systematic[sb] AND (mirtazapine) AND child	2
Search systematic[sb] AND (Memantine) AND child	3
Search systematic[sb] AND (Amantadine) AND child	27
Search systematic[sb] AND (Botulinum Toxin Type A) AND child	35
Search systematic[sb] AND (Montelukast) AND child	19
Search systematic[sb] AND (Simvastatin) AND child	5
Search systematic[sb] AND (cimetidine) AND child	2
Search systematic[sb] AND (Indomethacin) AND child	10
Search systematic[sb] AND (Flurbiprofen) AND child	0
Search systematic[sb] AND (Valproic acid) AND child	36
Search systematic[sb] AND (Divalproex) AND child	40
Search systematic[sb] AND (Topiramate) AND child	24
Search systematic[sb] AND (Eletriptan) AND child	1
Search systematic[sb] AND (Naratriptan) AND child	0
Search systematic[sb] AND (Pregabalin) AND child AND adverse	1
Search systematic[sb] AND (Levetiracetam) AND child AND adverse	4
Search systematic[sb] AND (amitriptyline) AND child AND adverse	6
Search systematic[sb] AND (carbamazepine) AND child AND adverse	28
Search systematic[sb] AND (Prochlorperazine) AND child AND adverse	2
Search systematic[sb] AND (melatonin) AND child AND adverse	7
Search systematic[sb] AND (melatonin) AND child	16
Search systematic[sb] AND (Naproxen) AND child	6
Search systematic[sb] AND (flunarizine) AND child	5
Search systematic[sb] AND (Dihydroergocryptine) AND child	0
Search systematic[sb] AND (dihydroergotamine) AND child	5
Search systematic[sb] AND (Ergotamine) AND child	1

March 29, 2012

#	Searches	Results
1	exp migraine disorders/dt	5944
2	exp migraine disorders/pc	1674
3	ad.fs.	991506
4	2 and 3	288
5	1 or 4	6107
6	1 or 2	7059
7	exp "off-label use"/	571
8	off label.mp.	2478
9	7 or 8	2478
10	6 and 9	14
11	exp calcium channel blockers/	68415
12	exp antihypertensive agents/	215895
13	exp antidepressive agents/	112330
14	exp anticonvulsants/	111378
15	exp botulinum toxin type a/	4780
16	exp alzheimer disease/dt	8048
17	11 or 12 or 13 or 14 or 15 or 16	474031
18	6 and 17	1675
19	5 or 10 or 18	6481
20	limit 19 to (humans and yr="2000 -Current")	3194
21	limit 20 to updaterange="mesz(20111121020154-20111121091315]"	0

Ovid Technologies, Inc. Email Service

Search for: limit 20 to (english language and "all child (0 to 18 years)")
Results: 100

Database: Ovid MEDLINE(R) <1946 to May Week 2 2012> Search Strategy:
----
1   exp migraine disorders/dt (5965)
2   exp migraine disorders/pc (1692)
3   ad.fs. (1002489)
4   2 and 3 (291)
5   1 or 4 (6136)
6   1 or 2 (7101)
7   exp "off-label use"/ (628)
8   off label.mp. (2572)
9   7 or 8 (2572)
10   6 and 9 (14)
11   exp calcium channel blockers/ (68722)
12   exp antihypertensive agents/ (217035)
13   exp antidepressive agents/ (113333)
14   exp anticonvulsants/ (112028)
15   exp botulinum toxin type a/ (4853)
16   exp alzheimer disease/dt (8211)
17   11 or 12 or 13 or 14 or 15 or 16 (477138)
18   6 and 17 (1689)
19   5 or 10 or 18 (6514)
20   limit 19 to (humans and yr="2000 -Current") (3226)
21   limit 20 to (english language and "all child (0 to 18 years)") (578)

Scientific Information Package requests and responses

Company Name	Date Responded
Abbott Laboratories	No response
Alexza Pharmaceuticals, Inc.	No response
Allergan, Inc.	No response
Almirall, S.A.	No response
AstraZeneca Pharmaceuticals, LP	No response
Beth Israel Deaconess Medical Center	No response
Boston Scientific	No response
BTG International, Ltd.	No response
Capnia, Inc.	No response
Centre Hospitalier Universitaire de Saint Etienne	No response
Cephalon, Inc	No response
Chengdu University of Traditional Chinese Medicine	No response
Clinvest	No response
CoLucid Pharmaceuticals, Inc.	No response
D-Pharm Ltd.	No response
Eisai Inc.	No response
Eli Lilly & Co	No response
Endo Pharmaceuticals	No response
eNeura	No response
Eurohead	No response
GlaxoSmithKline	Submitted
HaEmek Medical Center	No response
Ipsen Biopharm, Ltd	No response
Janssen Cilag Pharmaceutica S.A.C.I.	No response
Janssen EMEA	No response
Janssen Pharmaceutica NV	Submitted
Janssen-Ortho, Inc.	No response
Johnson & Johnson Pharmaceutical Research & Development, L.L.C.	No response
Kowa Pharmaceuticals America	No response
Lotus Pharmaceuticals, Inc.	No response
Luitpold Pharmaceuticals, Inc.	No response
Manhattan Pharmaceuticals, Inc.	No response
MAP Pharmaceuticals, Inc.	No response
Medtronic, Inc.	No response
Merck & Co., Inc.	Submitted
Nektar	Nothing to submit 11/16/2011
NeurAxon	No response
Nordlandssykehuset HF	No response
Novartis Pharmaceuticals Corporation	No response
NPS Pharmaceuticals	No response
Ortho-McNeil Janssen Scientific Affairs, LLC	No response
Ortho-McNeil Neurologics	No response
Ortho-McNeil-Janssen Pharmaceuticals, Inc	No response
Pfizer Inc	No response
Pozen	No response
PriCara® (Division of Ortho-McNeil-Janssen Pharmaceuticals, Inc.)	No response
Raptor Pharmaceutical Corp.	No response
Roxane Laboratories	No response
SK Chemicals	No response
Sorlandet Hospital HF	No response
Takeda Global Research & Development Center, Inc.	No response
Takeda Pharmaceuticals North America, Inc.	No response
The EMMES Corporation	No response
UCB, Inc.	No response
Valeant Pharmaceuticals International	No response
Zogenix	No response

Appendix B. Ongoing Studies of Migraine Prevention in Children

Appendix Table B1. Characteristics of ongoing studies of migraine prevention in children

Registration Number Recruitment	Interventions	Phases	Enrollment	Study Designs	Outcome Measures	Publication
NCT00195741 Completed	Drug: divalproex sodium	Phase 3	300	Allocation: Randomized|Endpoint Classification: Safety Study|Intervention Model: Parallel Assignment|Masking: Double-Blind|Primary Purpose: Treatment	Reduction from baseline in 4-week migraine headache rate|Migraine headache rate in last 4 weeks of study|Percent reduction from baseline|Percent of subjects with >75% reduction in migraine headache rate	Not available
NCT00195754 Completed	Drug: divalproex sodium	Phase 3	114	Allocation: Nonrandomized|Endpoint Classification: Safety Study|Intervention Model: Single Group Assignment|Masking: Open Label|Primary Purpose: Treatment	Safety outcome measure|Migraine headache rate	Not available
NCT00195806 Completed	Drug: divalproex sodium	Phase 3	315	Allocation: Nonrandomized|Endpoint Classification: Safety Study|Intervention Model: Single Group Assignment|Masking: Open Label|Primary Purpose: Treatment	Number of migraine headache days|Adverse events|Laboratory data|Vital signs|Study drug exposure|Behavioral/cognitive assessments	Not available
NCT00237302 Completed	Drug: topiramate	Phase 3	162	Allocation: Randomized|Endpoint Classification: Safety/Efficacy Study|Intervention Model: Parallel Assignment|Masking: Double-Blind|Primary Purpose: Prevention	Number of migraine days per month (28 days) during the double-blind treatment period relative to the prospective baseline period|Monthly rates of migraine episodes, nonmigraine headache episodes, and total headache days; percentage of treatment responders; severity and duration of migraines; frequency and severity of associated migraine symptoms, and use of rescue medicines.	Not available, but Clinical Study Report CR002662 is available with the outcomes and methods
NCT00210535 Completed	Drug: Topiramate; Placebo	Phase 3	110	Allocation: Randomized|Endpoint Classification: Safety/Efficacy Study|Intervention Model: Parallel Assignment|Masking: Double-Blind|Primary Purpose: Treatment	Percent reduction in the frequency of monthly migraine attacks (using 48-hour rule) over the last 12 weeks of the double-blind treatment phase compared with the 4-week prospective baseline period|Percent reduction in (a) average monthly migraine days, (b) average monthly headache days, and (c) monthly migraine rate, over the last 12 weeks of the double-blind treatment phase compared with the prospective baseline period.	Not available, but synopsis available (Clinical study report CR002245)

Registration Number Recruitment	Interventions	Phases	Enrollment	Study Designs	Outcome Measures	Publication
NCT00231595 Completed	Drug: topiramate	Phase 3	768	Allocation: Randomized|Endpoint Classification: Safety/Efficacy Study|Intervention Model: Parallel Assignment|Masking: Double-Blind|Primary Purpose: Treatment	Change in monthly (28 day) migraine period rate from the prospective baseline period to the double-blind phase.|Proportion of patients responding to the treatment. Changes from baseline to the double-blind phase in number of monthly migraine attacks, monthly migraine days, number of days/month requiring rescue medication and Health-Related Quality of Life measures	Brandes, 2004[1]
NCT00236509 Completed	Drug: topiramate	Phase 3	763	Allocation: Randomized|Endpoint Classification: Safety/Efficacy Study|Intervention Model: Parallel Assignment|Masking: Double-Blind|Primary Purpose: Treatment	Changes in length of time between the onset and cessation of painful migraine symptoms (migraine period) from baseline. Safety evaluations conducted throughout the study. Proportion of patients responding to the treatment. Changes from baseline to double-blind phase in number of monthly migraine attacks, monthly migraine days, number of days/month requiring rescue medication, and Health-Related Quality of Life measures.	Silverstein, 2004[2]
NCT00236561 Completed	Drug: topiramate, propranolol	Phase 3	786	Allocation: Randomized|Endpoint Classification: Safety/Efficacy Study|Intervention Model: Parallel Assignment|Masking: Double-Blind|Primary Purpose: Treatment	Change in the monthly (28 days) migraine period rate from the Prospective Baseline Period to the Core Double-Blind Phase. Proportion of patients responding to treatment. Change from Baseline Phase to Core Double-Blind Phase in number of monthly migraine attacks, monthly migraine days, number of days/month requiring rescue medication, and Health Related Quality of Life measures	Diener, 2004[3]
NCT00131443 Completed	Drug: Topiramate	Phase II|Phase III	40	Allocation: Randomized|Control: Dose Comparison|Endpoint Classification: Safety/Efficacy Study|Intervention Model: Parallel Assignment|Masking: Double-Blind|Primary Purpose: Educational/Counseling/Training	The primary efficacy outcome will be the reduction in average monthly migraine-days over the entire double-blind phase relative to the prospective baseline period|Reduction in frequency, severity and duration of basilar or hemiplegic aura symptoms|Reduction in migraine episode and headache episode frequency|Reduction in total headache days|Proportion of responders (i.e., the	Not available

Registration Number Recruitment	Interventions	Phases	Enrollment	Study Designs	Outcome Measures	Publication
					proportion of subjects who experience a ≥ 50% reduction in migraine-days and migraine episodes)|Cumulative reduction in frequency of migraine days and migraine episodes|Reduction in the use of acute/abortive medications|Reduction in migraine-associated symptoms	
NCT00158002 Completed	Drug: Topiramate	Phase II	40	Allocation: Nonrandomized|Control: Uncontrolled|Endpoint Classification: Safety/Efficacy Study|Intervention Model: Single Group Assignment|Masking: Open Label|Primary Purpose: Educational/Counseling/Training	Reduction of average monthly migraine days Reduction in frequency, severity and duration of basilar or hemiplegic aura symptoms|Reduction in migraine pain severity and duration|Migraine episode and headache episode frequency|Total headache days|Proportion of responders (i.e., the proportion of subjects who experience a 50% reduction in migraine-days and migraine episodes)|Cumulative frequency of migraine days and migraine episodes|Use of acute/abortive medications|Migraine episode and headache episode frequency|Total headache days|Migraine-associated symptoms	Not available
NCT00203255 Completed	Drug: Soy Isoflavones		25	Allocation: Nonrandomized|Control: Uncontrolled|Endpoint Classification: Efficacy Study|Intervention Model: Single Group Assignment|Masking: Open Label	To compare headache outcome measures between baseline and soy treatment periods. Headache outcome measures include frequency and duration of menstrually-associated migraine (MAM), as well as presence or absence of associated symptoms|Duration of MAM headaches|Maximum headache intensity|Incidence of MAM headache associated symptoms|Duration of MAM headache associated symptoms|Maximum functional impairment score during MAM headache|Incidence of use of rescue medication for the treatment of a MAM attack|Patient satisfaction score at the end of each treatment period|Describe headaches associated with menstruation|Describe the association of headache to premenstrual symptoms.|Explore premonitory	Not available

Registration Number Recruitment	Interventions	Phases	Enrollment	Study Designs	Outcome Measures	Publication
					symptoms in the menstrual migraine population|Compare questionnaire data collected at screening visit to questionnaire data collected at termination visit.|Assess electronic diary effectiveness in capturing diary information in this population	
NCT00475514 Completed	Drug: Frovatriptan 2.5mg QD|Drug: Frovatriptan 2.5 mg BID|Drug: placebo	Phase III		Allocation: Randomized|Control: Placebo Control|Intervention Model: Parallel Assignment|Masking: Double-Blind	Primary endpoint Number of MRM headache free PMPs out of a potential of three treated PMPs|Incidence of MRM headache|Maximum headache intensity|Incidence of moderate or severe MRM headaches|Number of MRM headache free days during treated PMPs|Incidence of MRM headache associated symptoms (e.g. photophobia, phonophobia, nausea and vomiting)|Functional impairment during treatment phase|Time to onset (days) of MRM headache (during the treated PMP and until five days post treatment)|Time to onset of first post-treatment migraine Incidence of intercurrent migraine outside of the peri-menstrual period Use of rescue medication	Not available
NCT00551980 Completed	Behavioral: Cognitive, Relaxation, Exercise Therapy	Phase III	2895	Allocation: Randomized|Control: Active Control|Endpoint Classification: Efficacy Study|Intervention Model: Parallel Assignment|Masking: Open Label|Primary Purpose: Treatment	Reduction in number of days per month with headache and shoulders pain after 6 months. Proportion of subjects with more than 4 days with headache and shoulder pain at the baseline that will have reduction in pain frequency of more than 50%, after 6 months|Headache index (Intensity x Frequency) after 6 and 12 months. Frequency of analgesic drug consumption after 6 and 12 months Frequency of headache and shoulder pain after 12 months	Not available
NCT01035983 Completed	Drug: Frovatriptan 2.5 mg	Phase III	550	Endpoint Classification: Safety Study|Intervention Model: Single Group Assignment|Masking: Open Label|Primary Purpose: Treatment	Incidence of all treatment-emergent adverse events (AEs).|Incidence of menstrual migraine headache|Maximum headache severity|Number of headache-free days during a treated perimenstrual period (PMP)|Occurrence and severity of menstrual migraine headache-	MacGregor, 2009[4]

Registration Number Recruitment	Interventions	Phases	Enrollment	Study Designs	Outcome Measures	Publication
					associated symptoms|Maximum functional impairment during menstrual migraine headache|Incidence and severity of intercurrent migraine|Total migraine burden|Standard hematology and biochemistry|12-lead electrocardiogram (ECG) and vital signs, physical examination|Short-form 12 (SF-12) Health Related Quality of Life Questionnaire	
NCT01581281 Not yet recruiting	Drug: Amitriptyline|Drug: Topiramate|Drug: Placebo	Phase 3	675	Allocation: Randomized|Endpoint Classification: Safety/Efficacy Study|Intervention Model: Parallel Assignment|Masking: Double Blind (Subject, Caregiver, Investigator, Outcomes Assessor)|Primary Purpose: Prevention	Reduction in Migraine Frequency (amitriptyline and topiramate)|Reduction in absolute migraine disability score on PedMIDAS|Safety and tolerability of amitriptyline and topiramate|Occurrence of treatment-emergent serious adverse events|Reduction in absolute migraine frequency days	Not available
NCT00269581 Active, not recruiting	Other: Educational CD-rom|Other: Headstrong CD-rom	Phase III	92	Allocation: Randomized|Control: Active Control|Endpoint Classification: Efficacy Study|Intervention Model: Parallel Assignment|Masking: Open Label|Primary Purpose: Treatment	Pain, mood, and stress self-rating scales|Quality of life|Headache-related disability	Not available
NCT00665236 Active, not recruiting	Other: Craniosacral therapy|Procedure: Low strength static magnets		66	Allocation: Randomized|Control: Placebo Control|Endpoint Classification: Efficacy Study|Intervention Model: Parallel Assignment|Masking: Single Blind (Outcomes Assessor)|Primary Purpose: Treatment	HIT-6|Headache frequency	Not available

References

1. Brandes JL, Saper JR, Diamond M, et al. Topiramate for migraine prevention: a randomized controlled trial. JAMA. 2004 Feb 25;291(8):965-73. PMID 14982912.
2. Silberstein SD, Neto W, Schmitt J, et al. Topiramate in migraine prevention: results of a large controlled trial. Arch Neurol. 2004 Apr;61(4):490-5. PMID 15096395.
3. Diener HC, Tfelt-Hansen P, Dahlof C, et al. Topiramate in migraine prophylaxis--results from a placebo-controlled trial with propranolol as an active control. J Neurol. 2004 Aug;251(8):943-50. PMID 15316798.
4. MacGregor EA, Brandes JL, Silberstein S, et al. Safety and tolerability of short-term preventive frovatriptan: a combined analysis. Headache. 2009 Oct;49(9):1298-314. PMID 19788471.

Appendix C. Analytical Framework

PICOTS Framework

Population(s)

Children with episodic migraine, chronic daily headache, or chronic migraine as defined by the Headache Classification Subcommittee of the International Headache Society[1] (see below for definitions).

Patient characteristics that can modify the effects of pharmacological treatments for preventing migraine attacks in children and adults:

- Age
- Sex
- The onset of menarche
- Race and ethnicity
- Socioeconomic status
- Education
- Family history
- Access to care, type of care, and residence in rural or urban areas
- Definition of migraine
- Presence of aura
- Headache frequency
- Prior treatments; overuse of drugs for acute migraine
- Obesity
- Nutritional and dietary factors, specifically caffeine
- Aerobic fitness
- Previous head injury
- Psychological factors and social/family support system
- Comorbidities (depression, bipolar disorder, anxiety, diabetes, hypertension, cardiovascular diseases, others)
- Concomitant medications for comorbid conditions

Interventions

Off-label medications previously examined in clinical trials for preventing migraine.[2]
Monotherapy.
Multidrug interventions.
Combined pharmacological with nonpharmacological modalities: behavioral interventions with education, exercise, biofeedback, relaxation techniques, yoga, massage, acupuncture, and dietary supplements.

Comparators

Placebo.
Drug treatments (comparative effectiveness).
Nonpharmacological treatments: behavioral interventions with education, exercise, biofeedback, relaxation techniques, yoga, massage, acupuncture, and dietary supplements.

Outcomes

Patient-centered outcomes:

Reduction of migraine attacks by >50 percent from baseline; primary outcome for the review.

Quality of life.

Patient satisfaction.

Composite patient centered outcomes defined as an aggregate improvement of the aforementioned outcomes.

Emergency visits, loss of school days; treatment failure.

Intermediate outcomes:

Number of headache days.

Number of moderate to severe headache days.

Improvement in associated symptoms.

Use of drugs for acute migraine (prescribed or over-counter).

Physician/healthcare professional (HCP) visits.

Harms:

All reported adverse reactions and effects (such as anxiety, nausea, vomiting, sleep time reduction, drowsiness, or weakness).

Treatment discontinuation due to adverse effects.

Additional medical resource utilization to manage adverse effects (e.g., prescription medication, urgent care/emergency services, physician/HCP visits).

Timing

6 months or more; optimally 12 months

Any time of occurrence for harms

Setting

Outpatient settings

Definition of Terms

Migraine (as defined by the Headache Classification Subcommittee of the International Headache Society):[1]

Repeated attacks of headache lasting 4 to 72 hours in patients with a normal physical examination, no other reasonable cause for the headache, and

At least two of the following features:

- Unilateral pain
- Throbbing pain
- Aggravation by movement
- Moderate or severe intensity

Plus at least one of the following features:

- Nausea/vomiting
- Photophobia and phonophobia

Episodic migraine as an indication for preventive treatment:

Five or more attacks a month[3]

Three or more attacks a month[3]

Definitions of chronic migraine (can be chronic from onset or transformed from episodic migraine):

FDA:

– Chronic migraine is defined as having a history of migraine and experiencing a headache on most days of the month.[4]

Revised International Headache Society criteria for chronic migraine:[1]

1.5.1. Chronic migraine

A. Headache (tension-type and/or migraine) on *≥15 days per month for at least 3 months*

* Characterization of a frequently recurring headache generally requires a headache diary to record information on pain and associated symptoms day by day for at least 1 month.

B. Occurring in a patient who has had at least five attacks.

C. On ≥8 days per month for at least 3 months headache has fulfilled C.1 and/or C.2 below; that is, has fulfilled criteria for pain and associated symptoms of migraine without aura.

1. Has at least two of a–d
   a. Unilateral location
   b. Pulsating quality
   c. Moderate or severe pain intensity
   d. Aggravation by or causing avoidance of routine physical activity (e.g., walking or climbing stairs) and at least one of (1) or (2):
      (1). Nausea and/or vomiting
      (2). Photophobia and phonophobia

2. Treated and relieved by triptan(s) or ergot before the expected development of C.1 above

D. No medication overuse† and not attributed to another causative disorder
   †Headache Classification Committee criteria for a medication overuse headache (A8.2)[1]

Diagnostic criteria for pediatric migraine without aura[5]

A. At least five attacks fulfilling criteria B through D

B. Headache attacks lasting 1 to 72 hours

C. Headache has at least two of the following characteristics:
   1. Unilateral location, which may be bilateral or frontotemporal (not occipital)
   2. Pulsing quality
   3. Moderate or severe pain intensity
   4. Aggravation by or causing avoidance of routine physical activity (e.g., walking, climbing stairs)

D. During the headache, at least one of the following:
   1. Nausea or vomiting
   2. Photophobia and phonophobia, which may be inferred from a child's behavior

E. Not attributed to another disorder

Diagnostic criteria for pediatric migraine with aura[5]—episodes of intense disabling headache separated by symptom-free intervals.

A. At least five distinct attacks lasting 1 to 72 hours and permit attacks to be briefer than in adults (range: 4–72 hours).
B. The location of the pain may be unilateral or, in children younger than 15 years of age, bilateral (bifrontal or bitemporal). The quality of pain is typically pulsing or throbbing, a symptom that may require specific questioning in young children.
C. The pain is moderate to intense and aggravated by routine physical activity, such as walking or climbing stairs.
D. The accompanying associated autonomic features (nausea, vomiting, photophobia, and phonophobia) may be as disabling as the pain. The latter two features may be inferred by the patient's behavior if the child withdraws to a quiet dark place during the attack.
E. The headache must be "not attributed to another disorder," implying that the prudent physician should carefully consider other possible causes for the recurrent headaches.

The disorders within the migraine with aura spectrum reflect the concept that the focal symptoms, such as visual disruptions, hemiparesis, and aphasia, are manifestations of the regional neuronal depolarization and oligemia caused by cortical spreading depression (CSD). Clinical entities of childhood with focal neurologic symptoms, previously termed *migraine variants*, such as hemiplegic and basilar type, now are included within this category of migraine with aura.

References

1. Olesen J, Bousser MG, Diener HC, et al. New appendix criteria open for a broader concept of chronic migraine. Cephalalgia. 2006 Jun;26(6):742-6. PMID 16686915.

2. Rapoport A. Antimigraine drugs: new frontiers. Neurol Sci. 2009 May;30 Suppl 1:S49-54. PMID 19415426.

3. Goadsby PJ, Raskin NH. Chapter 15. Headache. In: Fauci AS, Braunwald E, Kasper DL, Hauser SL, Longo DL, Jameson JL, et al., eds. Harrison's principles of internal medicine. 17th ed. New York: The McGraw-Hill Companies; 2008.

4. U.S. Food and Drug Administration. FDA News Release: FDA Approves Botox to Treat Chronic Migraine. http://www.fda.gov/NewsEvents/Newsroom/PressAnnouncements/ucm229782.htm. Accessed on February 1 2011.

5. Lewis DW. Pediatric migraine. Neurol Clin. 2009 May;27(2):481-501. PMID 19289227.

Appendix Table C1. Pharmacological classes for migraine prevention

Drug, ATC Code*	Class of Drug
ANTIEPILEPTICS	
Topiramate, N03AX11	N03 ANTIEPILEPTICS N03AX Other antiepileptics
Lamotrigine, N03AX09	N03A ANTIEPILEPTICS
Levetiracetam, N03AX14	N03A ANTIEPILEPTICS
Pregabalin, N03AX16	N03A ANTIEPILEPTICS alpha2-delta agonist
Carbamazepine , N03AF01	N03A ANTIEPILEPTICS N03AF Carboxamide derivatives
Valproic acid, N03AG01	N03A ANTIEPILEPTICS N03AG Fatty acid derivatives, Gamma-aminobutyric acid (GABA) enhancer and analog
Vigabatrin, N03AG04	N03A ANTIEPILEPTICS N03AG Fatty acid derivatives, GABA transaminase inhibitor
Tiagabine, N03AG06	N03A ANTIEPILEPTICS N03AG Fatty acid derivatives, gamma aminobutyric acid (GABA) enhancer
Zonisamide, N03AX15	N03A ANTIEPILEPTICS N03AX Other antiepileptics
Valproate	N03A ANTIEPILEPTICS N03AG Fatty acid derivatives
Divalproex	Gamma-aminobutyric acid (GABA) enhancer and analog
Gabapentin, N03AX12	N03A ANTIEPILEPTICS
Acetazolamide, S01EC01	S01EC, carbonic anhydrase inhibitor
ANTIDEPRESSANTS	
Nortriptyline , N06AA10	N06A ANTIDEPRESSANTS N06AA nonselective monoamine reuptake inhibitors
Clomipramine, N06AA04	N06A ANTIDEPRESSANTS N06AA nonselective monoamine reuptake inhibitors
Citalopram, N06AB04	N06A ANTIDEPRESSANTS N06AB Selective serotonin reuptake inhibitors
Venlafaxine, N06AX16	N06A ANTIDEPRESSANTS N06AX Other antidepressants
Amitriptyline	N06A ANTIDEPRESSANTS N06AA nonselective monoamine reuptake inhibitors
Mirtazapine, N06AX11	N06A ANTIDEPRESSANTS tricyclic antidepressants
BETA BLOCKERS	
Timolol, C07AA06	C07AA , Beta blocking agents, nonselective
Nadolol , C07AA12	C07AA Beta blocking agents, nonselective
Propranolol, C07AA05	C07AA Beta blocking agents, nonselective
Metoprolol, C07AB02	C07AB Beta blocking agents, selective
Atenolol, C07AB03	C07AB Beta blocking agents, selective
Bisoprolol, C07AB07	C07AB Beta blocking agents, selective
Acebutolol, C07AB04	C07AB Beta blocking agents, selective
Alprenolol, C07AA01	C07A BETA BLOCKING AGENTS
Oxprenolol, C07AA02 (discontinued in the FDA)	C07AA Beta blocking agents, nonselective
Pindolol, C07AA03	C07AA Beta blocking agents, nonselective
ACE INHIBITORS	
Trandolapril, C09AA10	C09AA ACE inhibitors
Enalapril, C09AA02	C09AA ACE inhibitors
Captopril, C09AA01	C09AA ACE inhibitors
Lisinopril, C09AA03	C09AA ACE inhibitors
ANGIOTENSIN II ANTAGONISTS	
Telmisartan, C09CA07	C09CA Angiotensin II antagonists
Candesartan, C09CA06	C09CA Angiotensin II antagonists
CALCIUM CHANNEL ANTAGONIST	
Dotarizine	SELECTIVE CALCIUM CHANNEL ANTAGONIST; 5-HT receptors ANTAGONIST
Flunarizine, N07CA03; Sibelium	SELECTIVE CALCIUM CHANNEL ANTAGONIST N07C ANTIVERTIGO PREPARATIONS

Drug, ATC Code*	Class of Drug
SELECTIVE CALCIUM CHANNEL BLOCKERS	
Nimodipine,C08CA06	C08C SELECTIVE CALCIUM CHANNEL BLOCKERS WITH MAINLY VASCULAR EFFECTS C08CA Dihydropyridine derivatives
Verapamil,C08DA01	C08D SELECTIVE CALCIUM CHANNEL BLOCKERS WITH DIRECT CARDIAC EFFECTS C08DA Phenylalkylamine derivatives
Nicardipine,C08CA04	C08C SELECTIVE CALCIUM CHANNEL BLOCKERS WITH MAINLY VASCULAR EFFECTS C08CA Dihydropyridine derivatives
Nifedipine,C08CA05	C08C SELECTIVE CALCIUM CHANNEL BLOCKERS WITH MAINLY VASCULAR EFFECTS C08CA Dihydropyridine derivatives
ANTIADRENERGICS	
Clonidine,C02AC01	C02A ANTIADRENERGIC AGENTS, CENTRALLY ACTING C02AC Imidazoline receptor agonists
Labetalol, C07AG01	C07AG , Alpha and beta blocking agents
Dixarit (clonidine, C02AC01) Guanfacine, C02AC02	C02A ANTIADRENERGIC AGENTS, CENTRALLY ACTING C02A ANTIADRENERGIC AGENTS, CENTRALLY ACTING C02AC Imidazoline receptor agonists
ANTI-DEMENTIA	
Donepezil, N06DA02 Memantine, N06DX01	N06 PSYCHOANALEPTICS N06D ANTI-DEMENTIA DRUGS N-methyl-D-aspartate (NMDA) receptor inhibitor
ANTIPSYCHOTICS	
Aripiprazole,N05AX12	N05A ANTIPSYCHOTICS
Olanzapine,N05AH03	N05A ANTIPSYCHOTICS N05AH Diazepines, oxazepines, thiazepines and oxepines
Quetiapine,N05AH04	N05A ANTIPSYCHOTICS N05AH Diazepines, oxazepines, thiazepines and oxepines
Deanxit (Flupentixol, N05AF01)	N05A ANTIPSYCHOTICS N05AF Thioxanthene derivatives
Sulpiride, N05AL01 (antipsychotic)	N05A ANTIPSYCHOTICS N05AL Benzamides
Prochlorperazine, N05AB04	N05A ANTIPSYCHOTICS
DOPAMINERGIC AGENTS	
Amantadine, N04BB01	N04B DOPAMINERGIC AGENTS N04BB Adamantane derivatives N-methyl-D-aspartate (NMDA) receptor inhibitor
Dihydroergocryptine, N04BC03	N04B DOPAMINERGIC AGENTS N04BC Dopamine agonists
ERGOT ALKALOIDS	
Dihydroergotamine, N02CA01	N02C ANTIMIGRAINE PREPARATIONS N02CA Ergot alkaloids
Lisuride, N02CA07 Ergotamine, N02CA02	N02C ANTIMIGRAINE PREPARATIONS N02C ANTIMIGRAINE PREPARATIONS N02CA Ergot alkaloids
Methysergide, N02CA04	N02C ANTIMIGRAINE PREPARATIONS N02CA Ergot alkaloids
MUSCLE RELAXANTS	
Botulinum Toxin Type A, M03AX01	M03A MUSCLE RELAXANTS, PERIPHERALLY ACTING AGENTS M03AX Other muscle relaxants, peripherally acting agents
Tizanidine, M03BX02	M03B MUSCLE RELAXANTS, CENTRALLY ACTING AGENTS
SYSTEMIC DRUGS	
Montelukast, R03DC03	R03D OTHER SYSTEMIC DRUGS FOR OBSTRUCTIVE AIRWAY DISEASES R03DC Leukotriene receptor antagonists

ATC code - The Anatomical Therapeutic Chemical classification

Appendix D. Evidence Tables

Table of Contents for Appendix D

Appendix Table D1. Characteristics of children in randomized controlled clinical trials about migraine prevention

Characteristics	Number of randomized trials that reported this information	Mean	Minimum	Maximum
Age	17	11.79	9.20	14.60
% females in sample	20	49.94	31.00	71.43
% Caucasians in sample	7	74.88	59.30	85.00
Duration of run in period in weeks	11	5.5	4.00	9.00
Headache frequency at baseline/month	16	8.39	3.20	17.30
Duration of migraine in years	6	3.58	2.20	4.70

Appendix Table D2. Reporting of characteristics of children in randomized controlled clinical trials about migraine prevention

Characteristics	Factor distribution	Number of trials	% of total
Migraine definition	Ad Hoc Committee	1	5.0
Migraine definition	Classic migraine	1	5.0
Migraine definition	International Headache Society	13	65.0
Migraine definition	Not specified	3	15.0
Migraine definition	Vahlquist's criteria	1	5.0
% of patients without aura	Not reported	13	65.0
Exclusion criteria	Not reported	6	30.0
Duration of migraine	Not reported	14	70.0
% preventative treatment	Not reported	19	95.0
Concurrent medication	Not reported	11	55.0
Prior treatment	Not reported	19	95.0
Overuse of the drugs for acute migraine	Not reported	20	100.0
Family factors	Not reported	15	75.0
Health insurance status of subjects	Not reported	19	95.0
Hormone therapy	Not reported	20	100.0
Inclusion of pregnant women/birth control	Not reported	18	90.0
Menses	Not reported	20	100.0
Obesity	Not reported	17	85.0
Socio-economic condition, education	Not reported	20	100.0
Subject compliance and suitability	Not reported	13	65.0
Definition of adherence to treatment	Not reported	15	75.0
Definition of adherence to treatment	Self-report	3	15.0
Definition of adherence to treatment	Tablet count	2	10.0

Appendix Table D3. Subject flow in randomized controlled clinical trials about migraine prevention in children

Treatments	Subject flow	Number of randomized trials that reported this information	Mean	Minimum	Maximum
All drugs	Number of screened potential subjects	3	338.7	46.0	504.0
All drugs	Number of enrolled subjects	9	115.67	15.0	436.0
All drugs	Total sample randomized to treatment	20	75.73	14.0	305.0
All drugs	% analyzed	16	94.95	73.6	100.0
All drugs	Number needed to screen	4	1.9	1.0	3.9
All drugs	Total length of followup	20	19.86	6.0	35.0
All drugs	Loss of followup in control group	7	8.72	3.3	24.7
All drugs	Loss of followup in active group	7	6.9	3.3	11.4
% analyzed	Topiramate	7	97.9	95.5	100.0
% analyzed	Divalproex	1	98.0	98.0	98.0
% analyzed	Valproate	0			
% analyzed	Trazodone	0			
% analyzed	Propranolol	4	85.3	73.6	95.2
% analyzed	Metoprolol	1	100.0	100.0	100.0
% analyzed	Clonidine	2	100.0	100.0	100.0
% analyzed	Magnesium	1	100.0	100.0	100.0
% analyzed	Internet	0			
Total length of followup	Topiramate	7	17.7	12.0	26.0
Total length of followup	Divalproex	1	12.0	-	-
Total length of followup	Valproate	1	12.0	-	-
Total length of followup	Trazodone	1	28.0	-	-
Total length of followup	Propranolol	4	27.8	24.0	35.0
Total length of followup	Metoprolol	1	32.0	-	-
Total length of followup	Clonidine	2	16.0	8	24
Total length of followup	Magnesium	1	16.0	-	-
Total length of followup	Internet	1	6.0	-	-
Loss of followup in control group	Topiramate	3	12.3	4.0	24.7
Loss of followup in control group	Divalproex	1	5.5	-	-
Loss of followup in control group	Valproate	0			
Loss of followup in control group	Trazodone	0			
Loss of followup in control group	Propranolol	2	4.4	3.3	5.5
Loss of followup in control group	Metoprolol	0			
Loss of followup in control group	Clonidine	1	9.8	9.8	9.8
Loss of followup in control group	Magnesium	0			
Loss of followup in control group	Internet	0			

Appendix Table D3. Subject flow in randomized controlled clinical trials about migraine prevention in children (continued)

Treatments	Subject flow	Number of randomized trials that reported this information	Mean	Minimum	Maximum
Loss of followup in active group	Topiramate	3	8.7	4.5	11.4
Loss of followup in active group	Divalproex	1	3.9	-	-
Loss of followup in active group	Valproate	0			
Loss of followup in active group	Trazodone	0			
Loss of followup in active group	Propranolol	2	4.2	3.3	5.1
Loss of followup in active group	Metoprolol	0			
Loss of followup in active group	Clonidine	1	9.8	9.8	9.8
Loss of followup in active group	Magnesium	0			

Appendix Table D4. Risk of bias in randomized controlled clinical trials about migraine prevention*

Risk of bias criteria	Distribution of criteria	Number of trials	% of total
Risk of bias	Low	12	50
Risk of bias	Medium	6	25
Risk of bias	Unclear	6	25
Masking of the treatment status	Double-blind	17	70.83
Masking of the treatment status	Not reported	6	25
Masking of the treatment status	Open-label	1	4.17
Intention to treat analysis preplanned	No	1	4.17
Intention to treat analysis preplanned	Not reported	11	45.83
Intention to treat analysis preplanned	Unclear	1	4.17
Intention to treat analysis preplanned	Yes	11	45.83
Allocation concealment	Adequate	5	20.8
Allocation concealment	Not adequate	1	4.17
Allocation concealment	Not reported	18	75

*Including flunarizine trials

Appendix Table D5. Risk of bias by journal of publication and funding of randomized controlled clinical trials about migraine prevention

Distribution factor	Low risk of bias	Medium risk of bias	Unclear risk of bias	Total	% of trials with low risk of bias
Total	9	6	5	20	45.0
Acta Neurol. Scandinav	1	0	0	1	100.0
Behaviour Research and Therapy	0	0	2	2	0.0
Development Medicine & Child Neurology	0	2	0	2	0.0
European Journal of Paediatric Neurology	0	0	1	1	0.0
Headache	6	3	0	9	66.7
Journal of Child Neurology	0	0	1	1	0.0
Pediatric Drugs	0	1	0	1	0.0
Pediatric Neurology	1	0	0	1	100.0
Pediatrics	1	0	1	2	50.0
Funding from Grant	1	1	2	4	25.0
Funding from Industry	5	2	0	7	71.4
No funding	0	1	1	2	0.0
Not reported	4	1	1	6	66.7
Other	1	0	0	1	100.0

Appendix Table D6. Randomized controlled clinical trials that examined efficacy of preventive drugs in children with migraine

Reference Design Sample Number analyzed % females	Age	Definition of migraine	Presence of aura	Baseline status	Overuse of drugs for acute migraine	Duration of migraine	Prior treatment	Subject compliance and suitability
Ludvigsson, 1974[1] Design RCT Sample 32 Number analyzed 28 43.75% female	Eligible age 7 to16 years Mean age Not reported	Ad hoc Committee on classification of headache 1962, Classification of headache, J.Amer.med. Ass., Bille 1962	4/32 had visual aura	Mean 3.4 attacks of headache per month	Not reported	4 years	Not reported	Not reported
Sillanpää, 1977[2] Design RCT Sample 57 Number analyzed 57 38.6% female	Eligible age 0-15 years Mean 11 years	Migraine was defined by the criteria of Vahlquist, i.e. paroxysmal headache separated by headache-free intervals and at least two of the following four: unilateral pain, nausea, visual aura and positive family history.	12 patients in the clonidine group and 8 patients in the placebo group had classic migraine with visual aura.	Frequency of headache/month(n): 1-2: Clonidine: 8, Placebo: 7, 3-4: Clonidine: 12 and Placebo: 12 , 5-6: Clonidine: 3 and Placebo: 4, and >6: Clonidine: 5 and Placebo: 6; Intensity of headache: Mild: Clonidine: 2 and Placebo: 0; Moderate: Clonidine: 6 and Placebo: 8 and Severe: Clonidine: 20 and Placebo: 19; Duration of headache: < hours: Clonidine: 6 and Placebo: 6, 4-6 hours: Clonidine: 9 and Placebo: 11 and >6 hours: Clonidine: 13 and Placebo: 11	Not reported	Not reported	Not reported	Not reported
Battistella, 1990[3] Design RCT Sample 37 Number analyzed Not reported 51.35% female	Eligible age 7 to 18 years Mean 12.2 years	Criteria of Ad Hoc Committee of the International Headache Society	9 patients had migraine with aura and 28 had migraine without aura	Frequency of attacks/month: Placebo: 3.0±0.9 and in Nimodipine: 3.3 ±0.9; duration (number of hours/attack):Placebo: 6.9±2.0 and in Nimodipine: 7.5±2.0	Not reported	Not reported	Prophylactic treatment was stopped for three months prior to the trial	Not reported

D-11

Appendix Table D6. Randomized controlled clinical trials that examined efficacy of preventive drugs in children with migraine (continued)

Reference Design Sample Number analyzed % females	Age	Definition of migraine	Presence of aura	Baseline status	Overuse of drugs for acute migraine	Duration of migraine	Prior treatment	Subject compliance and suitability
Battistella, 1993[4] Design RCT Sample 40 Number analyzed Not reported 45% female	Eligible age 7 to 18 years Mean 12.6 years	International Headache Society criteria for migraine	All patients had migraine without aura (inclusion criterion)	History of symptoms (yrs), mean (SD): 4.5 (1.3); mean frequency of attacks/month: Trazodone: 4.0±0.2 and Placebo: 3.5±0.1; Mean duration of attacks in hours: Trazodone: 20.2±1.3 and Placebo: 18.2±1.1	Not reported	4.5 years	Not reported	Not reported
Apostol, 2008[5] U.S. Food and Drug Administration, 2008[6] Design RCT Sample 305 Number analyzed 299 55% female	Eligible age 12 to 17 years Mean 14.2 years	International Headache Society criteria	Not reported	Migraine headaches within 3 months prior to screening: Mean (SD): Placebo: 16.7 (7.62), 250 mg DVPX ER: 16.6 (7.02), 500 mg DVPX ER: 18.0 (7.02), 1000 mg DVPX ER:17.3 (6.84)	Not reported	Not reported	Not reported	To document compliance with study medication, subjects were instructed to return all medication bottles and pill counts were performed. Site personnel were to counsel any subject with compliance <70%.
Lewis, 2009[7] Design RCT Sample 106 Number analyzed 103 61% female	Eligible age Between 12 and 17 years Mean 14.2 years	International Headache Society guidelines for pediatric migraine	Not reported	Mean migraine attacks, no/month: placebo: 4.1±1.48; 50mg topiramate: 4.1±1.74 and 100mg topiramate: 4.3±1.59 Mean migraine time: d/month: placebo: 6.1±3.02; 50mg topiramate: 6.4±2.86; and 100mg topiramate: 6.9±3.02	Not reported	Not reported	Not reported	Subjects maintained medication records the accuracy of which was checked by their parents.
Winner, 2005[8] Design RCT Sample 162 Number analyzed	Eligible age 6 to 15 years Mean 11.1	According to International Headache Society	Not reported	Mean (SD) monthly migraine days: topiramate: 5.4 (1.7) and placebo: 5.5 (2.0)	Not reported	Not reported	Not reported	Not reported

Appendix Table D6. Randomized controlled clinical trials that examined efficacy of preventive drugs in children with migraine (continued)

Reference Design Sample Number analyzed % females	Age	Definition of migraine	Presence of aura	Baseline status	Overuse of drugs for acute migraine	Duration of migraine	Prior treatment	Subject compliance and suitability
157 48.4% female	years	classification of pediatric migraine with or without aura						
Olness, 1987[9] Design RCT Sample 33 Number analyzed 28 39.3% female	Eligible age 6 to 12 years Mean 9.2 years	Classic migraine, defined as paroxysmal headache associated with all of the following: 1) unilateral head pain, 2) nausea/ vomiting, 3) visual aura (scotomas, visual field defects) or other transitory neurologic disturbance (sensory or motor), and 4) a history of migraine on one of the parents or a sibling.	All children had classic migraine.	Not reported	Not reported	Not reported	Not reported	Compliance was monitored by pill counts and maintenance of diaries

DVPX ER = Divalproex extended release; SD = standard deviation

D-13

Appendix Table D7. Ethical approval, funding, and conflict of interest in randomized controlled clinical trials that examined efficacy of preventive drugs in children with migraine

Reference Ethical approval Consent of participants	How project was funded Disclosure of conflict of interest Disclosed relationships
Ludvigsson, 1974[1] Ethical approval: Not reported Consent: Yes	Funding: Not reported Conflict of interest: Not reported
Sillanpää, 1977[2] Ethical approval: Not reported Consent: Not reported	Funding: Not reported Conflict of interest: Not reported
Sorge, 1985[10] Ethical approval: Not reported Consent: Not reported	Funding: Not reported Conflict of interest: Not reported
Battistella, 1990[3] Ethical approval: Not reported Consent: Not reported	Funding: Not reported Conflict of interest: Not reported
Battistella, 1993[4] Ethical approval: Not reported Consent: Not reported	Funding: Not reported Conflict of interest: Not reported
Apostol, 2008[5] U.S. Food and Drug Administration[6] Ethical approval: Yes Consent: Yes	Funding: Industry Conflict of interest: Not reported However, G. Apostol, G.A. Laforet, W.Z. Robieson, E. Olson, W.M .Abi-Saab, and M. Saltarelli are employees of Abbott, Abbott Park, IL,USA
Lewis, 2009[7] Ethical approval: Yes Consent: Yes	Funding: Grant Conflict of interest: Yes Dr Lewis received funds from Abbott Laboratories as a scientific advisor for study design and from Pfizer to attend a scientific advisory meeting in 2004 and received research grants from Abbott Laboratories, Astra Zeneca, Ortho-McNeil and Almirall. Dr Winner received funds from Merck, GlaxoSmithKline, Ortho-McNeil, Pfizer, Allergan, and Astra Zeneca for speaking, advisory board participation, and consultation and received research grants from GlaxoSmithKline, Ortho-McNeil, Pfizer, Allergan, Novartis, Wyeth, Merck, Forest Laboratories, Elan, Minster Pharmaceuticals, MAP Pharmaceuticals, Easai, and ReSearch Pharmaceutical Services. Dr Saper received speaking honoraria from GlaxoSmithKline, Merck, Ortho-McNeil, Neuralieve, Allergan, Medtronic, Pfizer, and Advanced Neuromodulation Systems and received research grants from Pfizer, Endo Pharmaceuticals, GlaxoSmithKline, Neuralieve, ProEthic, Ortho-McNeil, Johnson & Johnson, Merck, Alexa, Allergan, Cypress Pharmaceutical, Advanced Neuromodulation Systems, MAP Pharmacueticals, Medtronic, Torrey Pines Institute for Molecular Studies, and Schwarz Pharma. Drs Ness, Polverejan, Wang, Kurland, Nye, Yuen, Eerdekens, and Ford were employees of Johnson & Johnson.
Winner, 2005[8] Ethical approval: Yes Consent: Yes	Funding: Industry Conflict of interest: Not reported However, Ms Jordan, Dr. Fisher, and Dr .Hulihan are employees of Ortho-McNeil Pharmaceuticals, Raritan, NJ
Olness, 1987[9] Ethical approval: Yes Consent: Yes	Funding: Grant Conflict of interest: Not reported

Appendix Table D8. Risk of bias in randomized controlled clinical trials that examined efficacy of preventive drugs in children with migraine

Reference	Masking of the treatment status	Intention to treat analysis preplanned	Allocation concealment	Reporting of baseline data of the subjects	Adequacy of randomization	Selective outcome reporting	Risk of bias
Ludvigsson, 1974[1]	Double-blind	Not reported	Not reported	No	Not reported	Unclear	Low
Sillanpää, 1977[2]	Double-blind	Not reported	Not reported	Yes	Not reported	Unclear	Low
Sorge, 1985[10]	Double-blind	Not reported	Not reported	Yes	Yes	Unclear	Low
Battistella, 1990[3]	Double-blind	Not reported	Not reported	Yes	Yes	Unclear	Low
Battistella, 1993[4]	Double-blind	Not reported	Not reported	Yes	Not reported	Unclear	Low
Apostol, 2008[5]; The FDA review[6]	Double-blind	Yes	Unclear	Yes	Yes	Unclear	Low
Lewis, 2009[7]	Double-blind	Yes	Clearly adequate	Yes	Adequate	Unclear	Low
Winner, 2005[8]	Double-blind	Yes	Unclear	Yes	Not adequate. In the placebo group the % of white children was 87.8 and black children was 10.2, whereas in the topiramate group the % of white children was 72.2 and black children was 25.9		Medium
Olness, 1987[9]	Not reported	Not reported	Not reported	Yes	Yes	Unclear	Unclear

D-15

Appendix Table D9. Strength of evidence of reduction of baseline migraine frequency by >50% with antiepileptic topiramate in children (results from randomized controlled clinical trials)[7,8]

Dose	Rate, % Drug [placebo]	RCTs	Children	Directness	Risk of bias	Consistency	Precision	Dose response	Strength of evidence	Conclusion
100-200mg/day	61.2 [45.8]	2	230	Yes	Medium	Yes	Yes	Not applicable	Moderate	Topiramate, 100-200mg/day, did not increase rate of reduction in migraine by ≥50%
50mg/day	45.7 [45.5]	1	68	Yes	Low	NA	Yes	Not applicable	Low	Topiramate, 50mg/day, did not increase rate of reduction in migraine by ≥50%
50-200mg/day	58.2 [45.7]	2	298	Yes	Medium	Yes	Yes	No	Moderate	Topiramate, 50-200mg/day, did not increase rate of reduction in migraine by ≥50%

Appendix Table D10. Reduction in frequency of migraine attack by at least 50% from baseline with topiramate vs. placebo in children (pooled with random effects results from randomized controlled clinical trials)

Reference Dose of drug	Events/ randomized active	Events/ randomized control	Relative risk (95% CI)	Weight	Absolute risk difference (95% CI)	Weight	Risk of bias
100-200mg/day							
Winner, 2005[8] 50 mg/day at week 3, titrated to a max dose of 200 mg/day (2-3kg mg/kg/day)	61/112	23/50	1.18 (0.84 to 1.67)	39.71	0.09 (-0.08 to 0.25)	37.29	Medium
Lewis, 2009[7] 25mg/day initially and then gradually increased to 100mg/day, dosed twice daily *	29/35	15/33	1.82 (1.22 to 2.73)	34.41	0.37 (0.16 to 0.59)	32.65	Low
Pooled			1.45 (0.95 to 2.21)	74.12	0.22 (-0.06 to 0.51)	69.94	
50 mg/day							
Lewis, 2009[7] 25mg/day initially and then gradually increased to 50mg/day, dosed twice daily at the investigator's discretion	16/35	15/33	1.01 (0.60 to 1.69)	25.88	0.00 (-0.23 to 0.24)	30.06	Low
Pooled overall			1.32 (0.94 to 1.84)	100	0.15 (-0.06 to 0.37)	100	
Heterogeneity statistic			P value = 0.142 I squared = 48.7%		P value = 0.04 I squared = 68.8%		

*- at the investigator's discretion the dose was increased to the maximal dose tolerated by the subjects, 91% achieved the target daily dose during the double-blind treatment phase, the daily dose used during the entire double-blind treatment phase (titration and maintenance) was 73.6 ±18.7 mg/day

Appendix Table D11. Efficacy of topiramate on migraine prevention (results from a single RCT with medium risk of bias)[8]

Drug Dose	Definition of the outcome	Events/randomized with drug	Events/randomized with placebo	Relative risk (95% CI)	Absolute risk difference (95% CI)
Topiramate 50 mg/day at week 3, titrated to a max dose of 200 mg/day (2-3kg mg/kg/day)	≥75% reduction in monthly migraine days	36/112	7/50	**2.3 (1.1 to 4.8)**	**0.18 (0.05 to 0.31)**
	≥75% reduction in monthly migraine days during the last 28 days of treatment	57/112	15/50	**1.7 (1.1 to 2.7)**	**0.21 (0.05 to 0.37)**

Bold - significant difference at 95% confidence level when 95% CI of absolute risk difference do not include 0

D-18

Appendix Table D12. Reduction in migraine days with topiramate vs. placebo in children (pooled with random effects results from randomized controlled clinical trials)

Reference Dose of topiramate	Outcome with drug [Standard deviation]	Outcome with placebo [Standard deviation]	Standardized mean difference (95% CI)	Weight	Mean ratio (95% CI)	Weight	Risk of bias
Winner, 2005[8] 50 mg/day at week 3, titrated to a max dose of 200 mg/day (2-3kg mg/kg/day)	-2.6 [2.6]	-2.0 [3.1]	-0.22 (-0.55 to 0.12)	58.4	1.30 (0.81 to 2.08)	35.41	Medium
Lewis, 2009[7] 25mg/day initially and then gradually increased to 100mg/day, dosed twice daily *	-75.9 [32.42]	-49.7 [46.06]	-0.66 (-1.15 to -0.17)	41.6	**1.53 (1.08 to 2.16)**	64.59	Low
Pooled			-0.40 (-0.83 to 0.03)	100	**1.44 (1.09 to 1.91)**	100	
Lewis, 2009[7] 25mg/day initially and then gradually increased to 50mg/day, dosed twice daily at the investigator's discretion	-52.5 [48.55]	-49.7 [46.06]	-0.06 (-0.54 to 0.42)	100	1.06 (0.68 to 1.64)	100	Low
Pooled overall			-0.30 (-0.61 to 0.02)		**1.32 (1.04 to 1.67)**		Medium
Heterogeneity statistics			P value = 0.192 I squared = 39.4%		**P value = 0.434 I squared = 0%**		

Bold = significant difference at 95% confidence level when 95%CI of mean difference do not include 0; * - at the investigator's discretion the dose was increased to the maximal dose tolerated by the subjects, 91% achieved the target daily dose during the double-blind treatment phase, the daily dose used during the entire double-blind treatment phase (titration and maintenance) was 73.6 ±18.7 mg/day

Appendix Table D13. Strength of evidence of migraine prevention with antiepileptic divalproex sodium in children (results from a single randomized controlled clinical trial)[5]

Drug	Outcome	Dose	Rate, %	Children	Direct	Risk of bias	Consistency	Precision	Dose response	Strength of evidence	Conclusion
Divalproex sodium	Reduction of baseline headache frequency by ≥50%	250-1000 mg/day	40-50 [mean 45]	305	Yes	Low	Yes	Yes	No	Low	Divalproex sodium, 250-100mg/day did not increase rate of reduction in migraine by 50%

D-20

Appendix Table D14. Reduction in frequency of migraine attack by at least 50% from baseline with divalproex sodium vs. placebo in children (results from randomized controlled clinical trial with low risk of bias)[5]

Drug Dose	Definition of the outcome	Events/randomized with drug	Events/randomized with placebo	Relative risk (95% CI)	Absolute risk difference (95% CI)
Divalproex sodium 250mg once daily	≥50% reduction in 4 week migraine rate	33/83	33/73	0.9 (0.6 to 1.3)	-0.05 (-0.21 to 0.10)
Divalproex sodium 500mg once daily. For the first 2 weeks dose was 250mg/day	≥50% reduction in 4 week migraine headache rate	27/74	33/73	0.8 (0.5 to 1.2)	-0.09 (-0.25 to 0.07)
Divalproex sodium 1000 mg once daily. For the first 2 weeks dose was 500 mg/day	≥50% reduction in 4 week migraine headache rate	37/75	33/73	1.1 (0.8 to 1.5)	0.04 (-0.12 to 0.20)

Appendix Table D15. Reduction in migraine days with divalproex sodium vs. placebo in children (results from low risk of bias randomized controlled clinical trial)[5,6]

Reference Dose of divalproex sodium	Outcome with drug [Standard deviation]	Outcome with placebo [Standard deviation]	Mean difference (95% CI)	Standardized Cohen mean difference (95% CI)	Mean ratio (95% CI)
Apostol, 2008[5] U.S. Food and Drug Administration, 2008[6] 250mg once daily	-2.8 [2.91]	-2.8 [3.02]	0.0 (-0.9 to 0.9)	0.00 (-0.31 to 0.31)	1.00 (0.72 to 1.40)
Apostol, 2008[5] U.S. Food and Drug Administration, 2008[6] 500mg once daily. For the first 2 weeks dose was 250mg/day	-2.2 [3.18]	-2.8 [3.02]	0.6 (-0.4 to 1.6)	0.19 (-0.13 to 0.52)	0.79 (0.52 to 1.19)
Apostol, 2008[5] U.S. Food and Drug Administration, 2008[6] 1000 mg once daily. For the first 2 weeks dose was 500 mg/day	-3.1 [3.61]	-2.8 [3.02]	-0.3 (-1.4 to 0.8)	-0.09 (-0.41 to 0.23)	1.11 (0.77 to 1.59)

D-22

Appendix Table D16. Percentage of migraine headaches treated with symptomatic medications with divalproex sodium vs. placebo in children (individual low risk of bias randomized controlled clinical trial)[5]

Dose	Mean [Standard deviation] with drug, %	Mean [Standard deviation] with placebo, %	Mean difference, % (95% CI)	Cohen standardized mean difference (95% CI)	Means ratio (95% CI)
250mg once daily	-7.1 [34.0]	-9.7 [22.5]	2.6 (-6.3 to 11.5)	0.09 (-0.23 to 0.40)	0.73 (0.23 to 2.33)
500mg once daily. For the first 2 weeks dose was 250mg/day	-8.0 [29.6]	-9.7 [22.5]	1.7 (-6.8 to 10.2)	0.06 (-0.26 to 0.39)	0.82 (0.30 to 2.23)
1000 mg once daily. For the first 2 weeks dose was 500 mg/day	-8.5 [35.9]	-9.7 [22.5]	1.2 (-8.4 to 10.8)	0.04 (-0.28 to 0.36)	0.88 (0.29 to 2.61)

Appendix Table D17. Strength of evidence of migraine prevention with propranolol in children (results from randomized controlled clinical trials)

Outcome, Reference	Dose	Rate, % Drug [placebo]	RCTs	Children	Directness	Risk of bias Masking of treatment	Consistency	Precision	Dose response	Strength of evidence	Conclusion
Complete cessation of headache attacks Ludvigsson, 1974[1]	60mg-120mg/day	85 [14]	1	32, 28 analyzed	Yes	Low Double blind	Not applicable	Yes	Not applicable Large effect	Low	Propranolol Increased rates of complete cessation of headache attacks
Mean number of headaches Olness, 1987[9]	3mg/kg/d	Not applicable	1	33	Yes	Unclear Not reported	Not applicable	Yes	Not applicable	Insufficient	Propranolol did not decrease number of migraine days

Appendix Table D18. Reduction in frequency of migraine attack with propranolol vs. placebo in children (individual low risk of bias randomized controlled clinical trial)[1]

Dose	Definition of the outcome	Events/ randomized [rate, %] Propranolol	Events/ randomized [rate, %] Placebo	Relative risk (95% CI)	Absolute risk difference (95% CI)
Propranolol 60mg/day in three divided doses for children weighing less than 35 kg and 120mg/day in three divided doses for children weighing 35kg or more	Excellent degree of improvement before cross-over at 13 weeks (Excellent: No headache or only negligible symptoms remain)	9/13 [0.69]	1/15 [0.067]	**10.4 (1.5 to 71.4)**	**0.63 (0.34 to 0.91)**
	Excellent degree of improvement after cross-over at 26 weeks (Excellent: No headache or only negligible symptoms remain)	11/13 [0.85]	2/15 [0.14]	**6.3 (1.7 to 23.5)**	**0.71 (0.45 to 0.97)**
	Good degree of improvement before cross-over at 13 weeks (Good = Frequency of attacks reduced to <1/3 before cross-over at 13 weeks)	2/13 [0.154]	1/15 [0.07]	2.3(0.2 to 22.6)	0.09 (–0.15 to 0.32)
	Good degree of improvement after cross-over at 26 weeks (Good = Frequency of attacks reduced to <1/3)	1/13 [0.077]	0/15 [0]	3.4(0.2 to 77.6)	0.08 (–0.11 to 0.26)

Bold = significant improvement at 95% confidence level when 95% CI of absolute risk difference do not include 0

D-25

Appendix Table D19. Mean number of headaches per 3 month study period with propranolol vs. placebo in children (individual unclear risk of bias randomized controlled clinical trial)[9]

Dose	Mean [SD] with propranolol	Mean [SD] with placebo	Mean difference (95% CI)	Cohen standardized mean difference (95% CI)	Means ratio (95% CI)
3mg/kg/d in three divided doses	14.9 [12.9]	13.3 [9.5]	1.6 (−4.3 to 7.5)	0.14 (−0.38 to 0.67)	1.12 (0.74 to 1.70)

SD = Standard deviation

Appendix Table D20. Reduction in migraine days and duration with antidepressant trazodone vs. placebo (results from low risk of bias randomized controlled clinical trial)[4]

Definition of the outcome	Dose	Mean [SD] with drug	Mean [SD] with placebo	Mean difference (95% CI)	Cohen standardized mean difference (95% CI)	Mean ratio (95% CI)
Frequency of headache attacks/month	1mg/kg/day divided into 3 doses	2.8 [0.2]	1.2 [0.2]	**1.6 (1.5 to 1.7)**	**8.00 (6.10 to 9.90)**	2.33 (2.16 to 2.53)
Duration: number of hours/attack	1mg/kg/day divided into 3 doses	13.1 [1.3]	4.9 [0.7]	**8.2 (7.6 to 8.8)**	**7.85 (5.98 to 9.73)**	2.67 (2.48 to 2.89)

Bold = significant differences at 95% confidence level when 95% CI of mean difference do not include 0; SD = standard deviation

Appendix Table D21. Reduction in migraine days and duration with selective calcium channel blocker nimodipine vs. placebo (results from low risk of bias randomized controlled clinical trial)[3]

Dose	Definition of outcome	Mean [SD] with drug	Mean [SD] with placebo	Mean difference (95% CI)	Cohen standardized mean difference (95% CI)	Means ratio (95% CI)
10 to 20mg three times daily (<40kg to 10mg=5 drops TIS to 40-50 kg to 16mg=8 drops TID to >50kg to 20mg=10 drops TID)	Frequency of headache attacks/month	2.8 [0.6]	1.9 [0.7]	**0.9 (0.5 to 1.3)**	**1.38 (0.66 to 2.10)**	**1.47 (1.22 to 1.79)**
	Duration to number of hours/attacks	5.0 [1.2]	4.4 [1.1]	0.6 (-0.1 to 1.3)	0.52 (-0.13 to1.18)	1.14 (0.97 to 1.33)

Bold - significant differences at 95% confidence level when 95% CI of mean difference do not include 0; SD = standard deviation

Appendix Table D22. Strength of evidence of migraine prevention with clonidine, 25-50µg/day in children[2]

Outcome	Rate, % Drug [Placebo]	Children	Directness	Risk of bias	Consistency	Precision	Dose response	Strength of evidence	Conclusion
Reduction of baseline headache frequency	11 [24]	57	Yes	Low	NA	Yes	NA	Low	Clonidine did not increase rates of complete cessation or clinically important reduction of headache attacks
Reduction in acute drug utilization	50 [35]	57	Yes	Low	NA	Yes	NA	Low	Clonidine did not decrease acute drug utilization
Reduction in migraine severity	25 [14]	57	Yes	Low	NA	Yes	NA	Low	Clonidine did not decrease rate of mild migraine

Appendix Table D23. Reduction in frequency of migraine and severity with clonidine vs. placebo in children (results from individual double blind low risk of bias randomized controlled clinical trial)[2]

Dose	Definition of the outcome	Events/ Randomized	Events/ Randomized	Relative risk (95% CI)	Absolute risk difference (95% CI)
Clonidine 25µg once daily to children weighing 40kg or less and 25µg twice daily to those weighing more than 40kg	5-6: Headache frequency/month after treatment	2/28	0/29	5.2 (0.3 to 103.2)	0.07 (-0.04 to 0.18)
	Zero: Headache frequency/month after treatment	3/28	7/29	0.4 (0.1 to 1.5)	-0.13 (-0.33 to 0.06)
	1-2: Headache frequency/month after treatment	9/28	8/29	1.2 (0.5 to 2.6)	0.05 (-0.19 to 0.28)
	3-4: Headache frequency/month after treatment	6/28	4/29	1.6 (0.5 to 4.9)	0.08 (-0.12 to 0.27)
	Duration of headaches: >6 hours	6/28	5/29	1.2 (0.4 to 3.6)	0.04 (-0.16 to 0.25)
	Duration of headaches: 4-6 hours	5/28	2/29	2.6 (0.5 to 12.3)	0.11 (-0.06 to 0.28)
	Intensity of headache: moderate	7/28	5/29	1.5 (0.5 to 4.0)	0.08 (-0.13 to 0.29)
	Intensity of headache: severe	5/28	4/29	1.3 (0.4 to 4.3)	0.04 (-0.15 to 0.23)
	Intensity of headache: mild	7/28	4/29	1.8 (0.6 to 5.5)	0.11 (-0.09 to 0.32)
	Duration of headaches: <4 hours	6/28	6/29	1.0 (0.4 to 2.8)	0.01 (-0.20 to 0.22)
	Reduction for need for temporary drug therapy for single attacks	14/28	10/29	1.5 (0.8 to 2.7)	0.16 (-0.10 to 0.41)

Appendix Table D24. Randomized controlled clinical trials that examined comparative effectiveness of drugs for migraine prevention in children

Reference Total sample assigned to treatment Number analyzed % females	Question the study expects to answer	Age Definition of migraine Presence of aura	Baseline migraine status Comorbidity Concurrent medication Overuse of drugs for acute migraine	Duration of migraine Prior treatment Subject compliance and suitability
Ashrafi, 2005[11] Design RCT Sample 120 Number analyzed Not reported 33.9% females	To compare the effect of sodium valproate with that of propranolol in pediatric migraine prophylaxis	3 to 15 years 1988 International Headache Society criteria for pediatric common migraine All patients had migraine without aura	Mean headache frequency/month: sodium valproate: 7.8 and propranolol: 7.9 Not reported Not reported Not reported	Not reported Not reported Not reported
Bidabadi, 2010[12] Design RCT Sample 63 Number analyzed 60 33% females	To compare the efficacy and tolerability of propranolol and sodium valproate in the prevention of migraine in the pediatric population	5-15 years The diagnostic criteria for pediatric migraine without aura as defined by the International Headache Society. Not reported	Mean headache frequency per month: propranolol: 13.86 and sodium valproate: 13.23 Not reported Not reported Not reported	Not reported Not reported Monthly followup
Unalp, 2008[13] Design RCT Sample 48 Number analyzed 48 54.17% females	To compare the efficacy of topiramate and sodium valproate for the prevention of pediatric migraine	Not reported International Headache Society 2004 criteria for migraine headache Not reported	Duration of migraine episode, h: Sodium valproate: 10.2 (9.4), Topiramate: 7 (12); Headache frequency/month: Sodium valproate: 15.3 (10.1), Topiramate: 20.1 (10.2); Headache intensity, VAS: Sodium valproate: 6.8 (1) and Topiramate: 71 (1) Not reported Not reported Not reported	Not reported Not reported Not reported

D-31

Appendix Table D25. Funding and conflict of interest in randomized controlled clinical trials that examined comparative effectiveness of drugs for migraine prevention in children

Reference	Funding	Ethical approval of study	Consent of participants	Conflict of interest	Conflict of interests—relationship
Ashrafi, 2005[11]	Not reported	Not reported	Not reported	Not reported	Not applicable
Bidabadi, 2010[12]	None	Yes	Yes	None	Not applicable
Unalp, 2008[13]	No support	Yes	Not reported	None	Not applicable

Appendix Table D26. Risk of bias in randomized controlled clinical trials that examined comparative effectiveness of drugs for migraine prevention in children

Reference	Masking of the treatment status	Intention to treat analysis preplanned	Allocation concealment	Adequacy of randomization	Selective outcome reporting	Risk of bias
Ashrafi, 2005[11]	Not reported	Not reported	Not reported	Yes	Unclear	Unclear
Bidabadi, 2010[12]	Double-blind	No	Unclear	Yes	Unclear	Medium
Unalp, 2008[13]	Not reported	Not reported	Not reported	Yes	Unclear	Unclear

D-33

Appendix Table D27. Comparative effectiveness of sodium valproate vs. propranolol in preventing migraine in children (pooled with random effects models results from randomized controlled clinical trials)

Outcome	Reference Risk of bias	Active drug Dose vs. control drug, Dose	Events/randomized [rate of outcome in active group], %	Events/randomized [rate of outcome in control group], %	Relative risk (95% CI)	Weight	Absolute risk difference (95% CI)	Weight
Reduction in frequency of migraine attack by at least 50% from baseline	Ashrafi, 2005[11] Risk of bias Unclear	Sodium valproate,10-40mg/kg/day vs. Propranolol,1-3 mg/kg/day in two divided doses	43/60 [72]	41/60 [69]	1.0 (0.8 to 1.3)	54.62	0.03 (-0.13 to 0.20)	54.2
	Bidabadi, 2010[12] Risk of bias Medium	Sodium valproate,15 - 30mg/kg/day vs. Propranolol,2-3mg/kg/day	20/31 [64.5]	27/32 [84.4]	0.8 (0.6 to 1.0)	45.38	-0.20 (-0.41 to 0.01)	45.8
	P value=0.104 I squared=62.10%	Pooled	63/91 [69.5]	68/92 [74.4]	0.9 (0.7 to 1.2)	100	-0.07 (-0.30 to 0.15)	100
Complete cessation of headache attacks	Ashrafi, 2005[11] Risk of bias Unclear	Sodium valproate,10-40mg/kg/day vs. Propranolol,1-3 mg/kg/day in two divided doses	13/60 [21]	10/60 [17]	1.3 (0.6 to 2.7)	78.36	0.05 (-0.09 to 0.19)	54.81
	Bidabadi, 2010[12] Risk of bias Medium	Sodium valproate,15 - 30mg/kg/day vs. Propranolol,2-3mg/kg/day	3/31 [9.68]	4/32 [12.5]	0.8 (0.2 to 3.2)	21.64	-0.03 (-0.18 to 0.13)	45.19
	P value=0.5 I squared=0%	Pooled	16/91 [17.1]	14/92 [15.4]	1.2 (0.6 to 2.2)	100	0.02 (-0.09 to 0.12)	100

D-34

Appendix Table D28. Comparative effectiveness of sodium valproate vs. propranolol in preventing migraine in children (results from individual randomized controlled clinical trials)

Definition of the outcome	Active vs. control drug	Reference Risk of bias	Events/randomized in active Control group Rate in active [control] group, %	Relative risk (95% CI)	Absolute risk difference (95% CI)
Reduction of headache severity by at least one grade	Sodium valproate, 15-30mg/kg/day vs. Propranolol, 2-3mg/kg/day	Bidabadi, 2010[12] Risk of bias: Medium	17/31 20/32 54.8 [62.5]	0.9 (0.6 to 1.3)	-0.08 (-0.32 to 0.17)
Reduction of headache duration	Sodium valproate, 10-40mg/kg/day vs. Propranolol, 1-3 mg/kg/day in two divided doses	Ashrafi, 2005[11] Risk of bias: Unclear	31/60 32/60 52.0 [53.0]	1.0 (0.7 to 1.4)	-0.02 (-0.20 to 0.16)
Reduction of baseline headache frequency by >70%	Sodium valproate,15-30mg/kg/day vs. Propranolol, 2-3mg/kg/day	Bidabadi, 2010[12] Risk of bias: Medium	10/31 21/32 32.3 [65.6]	**0.5 (0.3 to 0.9)**	**-0.33 (-0.57 to -0.10)**
Reduction of baseline headache frequency by 50-70%	Sodium valproate, 15-30mg/kg/day vs. Propranolol, 2-3mg/kg/day	Bidabadi, 2010[12] Risk of bias: Medium	9/31 4/32 29.0 [12.5]	2.3 (0.8 to 6.8)	0.17 (-0.03 to 0.36)
Better response to rescue medications	Sodium valproate, 10-40mg/kg/day vs. Propranolol, 1-3 mg/kg/day in two divided doses	Ashrafi, 2005[11] Risk of bias: Unclear	37/60 40/60 61.0 [67.0]	0.9 (0.7 to 1.2)	-0.05 (-0.22 to 0.12)
Reduction of baseline headache frequency by 20-50%	Sodium valproate,15-30mg/kg/day vs. Propranolol, 2-3mg/kg/day	Bidabadi, 2010[12] Risk of bias: Medium	7/31 3/32 22.6 [9.4]	2.4 (0.7 to 8.5)	0.13 (-0.05 to 0.31)
Reduction of baseline headache frequency by <20%	Sodium valproate,15-30mg/kg/day vs. Propranolol, 2-3mg/kg/day	Bidabadi, 2010[12] Risk of bias: Medium	4/31 2/32 12.9 [6.3]	2.1 (0.4 to 10.5)	0.07 (-0.08 to 0.21)
Reduction of headache severity at least for one grade	Sodium valproate, 10-40mg/kg/day vs. Propranolol, 1-3 mg/kg/day in two divided doses	Ashrafi, 2005[11] Risk of bias: Unclear	34/60 38/60 56.0 [64.0]	0.9 (0.7 to 1.2)	-0.07 (-0.24 to 0.11)

Bold = significant differences at 95% confidence level when 95% CI of absolute risk difference do not include 0

Appendix Table D29. Comparative effectiveness of topiramate vs. sodium valproate in preventing migraine in children (results from a randomized controlled clinical trial)[13]

Definition of the outcome	Active vs. control drug	Level of outcome [SD] /number of subjects in active group and control group	Mean difference (95% CI)	Cohen standardized mean difference (95% CI)	Means Ratio (95%CI)
Headache frequency/month: After therapy	Topiramate, 1-3mg/kg vs. sodium valproate, 10-15mg/kg	4.4 [5.5]/28 5.5 [6.6]/20	-2.20 (-6.48 to 2.08)	-0.32 (-0.89 to 0.26)	0.67 (0.32 to 1.39)
Headache intensity (VAS): After therapy	Topiramate, 1-3mg/kg vs. sodium valproate, 10-15mg/kg	3.2 [1.8]/28 1.8 [3.4]/20	-0.20 (-1.34 to 0.94)	-0.10 (-0.68 to 0.47)	0.94 (0.67 to 1.32)
Duration of migraine episode (h)	Topiramate, 1-3mg/kg vs. sodium valproate, 10-15mg/kg	2.4 [3.1]/28 3.1 [1.4]/20	1.00 (-0.59 to 2.59)	0.35 (-0.23 to 0.93)	1.71 (0.69 to 4.29)
PedMIDAS (Pediatric Migraine Disability Assessment Score)	Topiramate, 1-3mg/kg vs. sodium valproate, 10-15mg/kg	4.6 [6.5]/28 6.5 [5.5]/20	-0.90 (-5.60 to 3.80)	-0.12 (-0.69 to 0.46)	0.84 (0.34 to 2.06)

SD = Standard deviation

Appendix Table D30. Randomized controlled clinical trials that examined comparative effectiveness of drugs vs. active nonpharmacologic treatments for migraine prevention in children

Reference Design Sample Analyzed % female	Aim	Age	Definition of migraine	Presence of aura	Baseline status of subjects: disease	Duration of migraine	Subject compliance and suitability
Olness, 1987[9] Design RCT Sample 33 Number of analyzed 28 39.3% female	Propranolol, vs. self-hypnosis	6-12 years Mean 9.2 years	Classic migraine.	All children had classic migraine	Not reported	Not reported	Compliance was monitored by pill counts and maintenance of dairies
Sartory, 1998[14] Design RCT Sample 43 Number of analyzed 43 39.5% female	Metoprolol vs. progressive relaxation training and vasomotor feedback	8-16 years Mean 11.3 years	IHS criteria	16 37.2% children had migraine with aura	Headache frequency/week: relaxation group: 2.24 (1.89), vasomotor feedback group: 1.77 (1.17), and metoprolol group: 1.33 (0.62)	4.7 years	Not reported

Appendix Table D31. Funding and conflict of interest in randomized controlled clinical trials that examined comparative effectiveness of drugs vs. active nonpharmacologic treatments for migraine prevention in children

Reference	How project was funded	Ethical approval of study	Consent of participants	Conflict of interest	Conflict of interests-relationship
Olness, 1987[9]	Grant	Yes	Yes	Not reported	Not applicable
Sartory, 1998[14]	Other	Not reported	Yes	Not reported	Not applicable

Appendix Table D32. Risk of bias in randomized controlled clinical trials that examined comparative effectiveness of drugs vs. active nonpharmacologic treatments for migraine prevention in children

Reference	Masking of the treatment status	Intention to treat analysis preplanned	Allocation concealment	Reporting of baseline data of subjects	Adequacy of randomization	Selective outcome reporting	Risk of bias
Olness, 1987[9]	Not reported	Not reported	Not reported	Yes	Yes	Unclear	Unclear
Sartory, 1998[14]	Not reported	Not reported	Unclear	Yes	Not adequate	Unclear	Unclear

Appendix Table D33. Comparative effectiveness of metoprolol and nonpharmacologic treatments in unclear risk of bias randomized controlled clinical trial[14]

Active drug and dose	Nonpharmacological treatment	Definition of the outcome	Events/randomized in active and control Rate of outcome in active [control], %	Relative risk (95% CI)	Absolute risk difference (95% CI)
Metoprolol 50mg once daily in children <40kg body weight and 100mg in children >40kg. During first week of treatment half of this dose was given.	Progressive relaxation training + stress management	Percentage of patients who improved by more than 50% in the headache index (percent change from baseline to post-treatment of frequency *intensity of headache episodes)	5/13 12/15 38.5 [80.0]	0.5 (0.2 to 1.0)	-0.42 (-0.75 to -0.08)
Metoprolol 50mg once daily in children <40kg body weight and 100mg in children >40kg. During first week of treatment half of this dose was given.	Cephalic vasomotor feedback + stress management	Percentage of patients who improved by more than 50% in the headache index (percent change from baseline to post-treatment of frequency *intensity of headache episodes)	5/13 8/15 38.5 [53.3]	0.7 (0.3 to 1.7)	-0.15 (-0.51 to 0.22)

Appendix Table D34. Comparative effectiveness of metoprolol and nonpharmacologic treatments in unclear risk of bias randomized controlled clinical trial, mean differences[14]

Active drug and dose	Nonpharmacological treatment	Definition of the outcome	Mean [standard deviation] with drug	Mean [standard deviation] with nondrug	Mean difference (95% CI)	Cohen standardized mean difference (95% CI)	Means ratio (95% CI)
Metoprolol 50mg once daily in children <40kg body weight and 100mg in children >40kg. During first week of treatment half his dose was given.	Progressive relaxation training + stress management	Frequency of headache at 8 month followup	1.25 [0.82]	1.14 [1.19]	0.11 (-0.64 to 0.86)	0.11 (-0.64 to 0.85)	1.10 (0.58 to 2.07)
Metoprolol 50mg once daily in children <40kg body weight and 100mg in children >40kg. During first week of treatment half his dose was given.	Progressive relaxation training + stress management	Frequency of headache at 8 month followup	1.25 [0.82]	1.05 [0.72]	0.20 (-0.38 to 0.78)	0.26 (-0.49 to 1.01)	1.19 (0.72 to 1.96)
Metoprolol 50mg once daily in children <40kg body weight and 100mg in children >40kg. During first week of treatment half his dose was given.	Progressive relaxation training + stress management	Intensity of headache at 8 month followup (intensity was measured on a scale of 1 (light) to 10 (overbearing))	4.19 [2.42]	3.09 [1.67]	1.10 (-0.46 to 2.66)	0.54 (-0.22 to 1.29)	1.36 (0.89 to 2.06)
Metoprolol 50mg once daily in children <40kg body weight and 100mg in children >40kg. During first week of treatment half his dose was given.	Progressive relaxation training + stress management	Intensity of headache at 8 month followup (intensity was measured on a scale of 1 (light) to 10 (overbearing))	4.19 [2.42]	2.98 [2.65]	1.21 (-0.67 to 3.09)	0.48 (-0.28 to 1.23)	1.41 (0.81 to 2.43)

Appendix Table D35. Comparative effectiveness of propranolol and self-hypnosis in unclear risk of bias randomized controlled clinical trial[9]

Active drug and dose	Nonpharmacological treatment	Definition of the outcome	Mean [Standard deviation] with drug	Mean [Standard deviation] with nondrug	Mean difference (95% CI)	Cohen standardized mean difference (95% CI)	Means ratio (95%CI)
Propranolol 3mg/kg/d in three divided doses	Self-hypnosis	Mean number of headaches per 3 month study period	14.90 [12.9]	5.80 [5.8]	**9.10 (3.86 to 14.34)**	**0.91 (0.36 to 1.46)**	**2.57 (1.57 to 4.19)**

Bold = significant differences when 95% CI of mean difference do not include 0

Appendix Table D36. Randomized controlled clinical trials that examined dose response effectiveness of drugs for migraine prevention in children

Reference Sample Total number analyzed % females	Eligible age Mean age	Definition of migraine	Presence of aura	Baseline status of subjects: disease	Duration of migraine
Winner, 2006[15] Sample 51 Number analyzed 49 71% females	Eligible age 12-17 years Mean age 14 years	International Headache Society criteria	Not reported	Migraine frequency, Mean (SD): Topiramate 50mg/day: 4.8 (1.9), Topiramate 100mg/day: 6.2 (3.5), Topiramate 200mg/day: 4.9 (2.0);	Not reported
Lewis, 2007[16] Sample 14 Number analyzed 14 71.43% females	Eligible age 6 to 18 years Mean age 13.43 years	According to ICHD-2 criteria for basilar migraine	100% of patients had aura; 8 of 14 patients also had periodic attacks of migraine without aura	Average number of migraines per month, median: 25mg group: 8 and 100mg/d group: 5 ; Average severity of migraine, mean (SD), 0-5 point scale: 25mg group: 3.37 (0.53) and 100mg group: 3.4 (0.67)	4.2 years
Lewis, 2009[7], Pandina, 2010[17] Sample 103 Number analyzed 103 61% females	Eligible age 12-17 years Mean age 14.2 years	International Headache Society criteria for pediatric migraine	Not reported	Mean migraine attacks, no/month: placebo: 4.1±1.48: 50mg topiramate: 4.1±1.74 and 100mg topiramate: 4.3±1.59 Mean migraine time: d/month: placebo: 6.1±3.02: 50mg topiramate: 6.4±2.86; and 100mg topiramate: 6.9±3.02	Not reported
Apostol, 2008[5] U.S. Food and Drug Administration, 2008[6] Sample 305 Number analyzed 299 55% females	Eligible age 12-17 years Mean age 14.2 years	International Headache Society criteria	Not reported	Migraine headaches within 3 months prior to screening: Mean (SD):Placebo: 16.7 (7.62), 250 mg DVPX ER: 16.6 (7.02), 500 mg DVPX ER: 18.0 (7.02), 1000 mg DVPX ER:17.3 (6.84)	Not reported

SD = Standard deviation

Appendix Table D37. Funding and conflict of interest in randomized controlled clinical trials that examined dose response effectiveness of drugs for migraine prevention in children

Reference	How project was funded	Ethical approval of study	Consent of participants	Conflict of interest	Conflict of interest—relationship
Winner, 2006[15]	Industry	Yes	Yes	Yes	Drs. Winner and Gendolla have received consulting and speaker fees from Johnson & Johnson. Drs. Stayer, Wang, Yuen, Battisti, and Nye are employees of the company.
Lewis, 2007[16]	Industry	Yes	Yes	Yes	The study was supported by a research grant from Ortho-McNeil Neurologies Inc. as an investigator-initiated project.
Apostol, 2008[5] U.S. Food and Drug Administration, 2008[6]	Industry	Yes	Yes	Not reported	Not reported, however, G. Apostol, G.A. Laforet, W.Z. Robieson, E. Olson, W.M. Abi-Saab, and M. Saltarelli are employees of Abbott, Abbott Park, IL, USA
Lewis, 2009[7]	Grant	Yes	Yes	Yes	Dr. Lewis received funds from Abbott Laboratories as a scientific advisor for study design and from Pfizer to attend a scientific advisory meeting in 2004 and received research grants from Abbott Laboratories, Astra Zeneca, Ortho-McNeil and Almirall. Dr Winner received funds from Merck, GlaxoSmithKline, Ortho-McNeil, Pfizer, Allergan, and Astra Zeneca for speaking, advisory board participation, and consultation and received research grants from GlaxoSmithKline, Ortho-McNeil, Pfizer, Allergan, Novartis, Wyeth, Merck, Forest Laboratories, Elan, Minster Pharmaceuticals, MAP Pharmaceuticals, Easai, and ReSearch Pharmaceutical Services. Dr. Saper received speaking honoraria from GlaxoSmithKline, Merck, Ortho-McNeil, Neuralieve, Allergan, Medtronic, Pfizer, and Advanced Neuromodulation Systems and received research grants from Pfizer, Endo Pharmaceuticals, GlaxoSmithKline, Neuralieve, ProEthic, Ortho-McNeil, Johnson & Johnson, Merck, Alexa, Allergan, Cypress Pharmaceutical, Advanced Neuromodulation Systems, MAP Pharmacueticals, Medtronic, Torrey Pines Institute for Molecular Studies, and Schwarz Pharma. Drs Ness, Polverejan, Wang, Kurland, Nye, Yuen, Eerdekens, and Ford were employees of Johnson & Johnson.
Pandina, 2010[17]	Industry	Yes	Yes	Yes	George Rogan MS, of Phase Five Communications, Inc. helped to coordinate, edit, and finalize the manuscript for submission

D-44

Appendix Table D38. Risk of bias in randomized controlled clinical trials that examined dose response effectiveness of drugs for migraine prevention in children

Reference	Masking of treatment status	Intention to treat analysis preplanned	Allocation concealment	Adequacy of randomization	Selective outcome reporting	Risk of bias
Winner, 2006[15]	Double-blind	Yes	Clearly adequate (computer-generated randomization schedule)	Not adequate (Topiramate 100mg had higher mean frequency and days of migraine compared to other groups and topiramate 200mg had higher percentage of men and women compared to other groups)	Unclear	Low
Lewis, 2007[16]	Double-blind	Yes	Unclear	Adequate	Unclear	Low
Apostol, 2008[5] U.S. Food and Drug Administration, 2008[6]	Double-blind	Yes	Unclear	Adequate	Unclear	Low
Lewis, 2009[7]	Double-blind	Yes	Clearly adequate	Adequate	Unclear	Low
Pandina, 2010[17]	Double-blind	Yes	Not reported	Adequate	Unclear	Low

D-45

Appendix Table D39. Dose response effects with topiramate in preventing migraine in children (results from randomized controlled clinical trials)

Compared daily doses	Outcomes	Reference	Events/ randomized with higher dose	Events/ randomized with lower dose	Relative risk (95% CI)	Absolute risk difference 95% CI)
Topiramate 25mg vs. 100mg	Overall Parent Global Assessment: Much improved	Lewis, 2007[16]	2/7	0/7	5.0 (0.3to 88.5)	0.29(-0.08 to 0.65)
	Overall Parent Global Assessment: Very much improved	Lewis, 2007[16]	4/7	3/7	1.3 (0.5to 3.9)	0.14(-0.38 to 0.66)
	Overall Parent Global Assessment: Minimally improved	Lewis, 2007[16]	0/7	1/7	0.3 (0.0 to 7.0)	-0.14(-0.46 to 0.18)
	Overall Parent Global Assessment: No change	Lewis, 2007[16]	1/7	2/7	0.5 (0.1 to 4.3)	-0.14(-0.57 to 0.28)
	Greater than 50% reduction in migraine frequency	Lewis, 2007[16]	7/7	5/7	1.4 (0.8 to 2.2)	0.29(-0.08 to 0.65)
Topiramate 50mg vs. 100mg	Responder, that is, ≥50% reduction in the monthly migraine attack rate	Lewis, 2009[*]	16/35	29/35	**0.6 (0.4 to 0.8)**	**-0.37(-0.58 to -0.16)**

Bold = significant difference at 95% confidence level when 95% CI of absolute risk difference do not include 0; * at the investigator's discretion the dose was increased to the maximal dose tolerated by the subjects, 91% achieved the target daily dose during the double-blind treatment phase, the daily dose used during the entire double-blind treatment phase (titration and maintenance) was 73.6 ±18.7 mg/day

Appendix Table D40. Dose response reduction in migraine intermediate outcomes with topiramate in children, results from randomized controlled clinical trials[16]

Compared doses, references	Outcome	Mean [Standard deviation] with higher dose	Mean [Standard deviation] with lower dose	Mean difference (95% CI)	Cohen standardized mean difference (95% CI)
Topiramate 25mg vs. 100mg[16]	Difference in PedMIDAS score of headache disability: grade I is 0-10 (none to mild) to grade IV is >50 (severe).	-35.1 [22.4]	-23.3 [28.3]	-11.85 (-38.59 to 14.89)	-0.46 (-1.53 to 0.60)
Topiramate 25mg vs. 100mg[16]	Difference in average monthly basilar migraine days from baseline	-3.0 [2.5]	-1.9 [2.8]	-1.03 (-3.76 to 1.70)	-0.39 (-1.45 to 0.66)
Topiramate 50mg vs. 100mg[7]*	Mean percent reduction in migraine day rate	-52.1 [58.6]	-73.3 [37.8]	21.20 (-1.90 to 44.30)	0.43 (-0.04 to 0.90)
Topiramate 50mg vs. 100mg[7]*	Last 4 week of double-phase: migraine attacks, number per month	1.9 [2.0]	1.1 [1.5]	0.80 (-0.02 to 1.62)	0.46 (-0.02 to 0.93)
Topiramate 50mg vs. 100mg[7]*	**Mean percent reduction in migraine day rate**	**-52.5 [48.6]**	**-75.9 [32.4]**	**23.40 (4.06 to 42.74)**	**0.57 (0.09 to 1.04)**
Topiramate 50mg vs. 100mg[7]*	Mean migraine time, days/month (last 4 weeks of double-blind phase)	2.8 [3.3]	2.0 [2.9]	0.80 (-0.65 to 2.25)	0.26 (-0.21 to 0.73)

Bold = significant difference at 95% confidence level when 95% CI of mean difference do not include 0; * - at the investigator's discretion the dose was increased to the maximal dose tolerated by the subjects, 91% achieved the target daily dose during the double-blind treatment phase, the daily dose used during the entire double-blind treatment phase (titration and maintenance) was 73.6 ±18.7 mg/day

Appendix Table D41. Dose response effects with divalproex sodium in preventing migraine in children (results from low risk of bias randomized controlled clinical trial)[5]

Compared doses	Outcome	Events/ randomized with higher dose	Events/ randomized with lower dose	Relative risk (95% CI)	Absolute risk difference 95% CI)
Divalproex sodium 250mg vs. 500mg	≥50% reduction in 4 week migraine headache rate	33/83	27/74	1.1 (0.7 to 1.6)	0.03 (-0.12 to 0.18)
Divalproex sodium 250mg vs. 1000mg	≥50% reduction in 4 week migraine headache rate	33/83	37/75	0.8 (0.6 to 1.1)	-0.10 (-0.25 to 0.06)
Divalproex sodium 500mg vs. 1000mg	≥50% reduction in 4 week migraine headache rate	27/74	37/75	0.7 (0.5 to 1.1)	-0.13 (-0.29 to 0.03)

Appendix Table D42. Dose response reduction in migraine intermediate outcomes with divalproex sodium in children (results from randomized controlled clinical trial)[5,6]

Compared doses	Outcome	Mean [Standard deviation] with higher dose	Mean [Standard deviation] with lower dose	Mean difference (95% CI)	Cohen standardized mean difference (95% CI)
Divalproex sodium 250mg vs. 500mg	Migraine headache rate: Reduction from baseline, last 4 weeks	-1.7 [1.8]	-2.0 [1.8]	0.30 (-0.28 to 0.88)	0.16 (-0.15 to 0.48)
Divalproex sodium 250mg vs. 500mg	Migraine headache rate: experimental phase % reduction from baseline	-33.1 [56.2]	-36.3 [36.9]	3.20 (-11.52 to 17.92)	0.07 (-0.25 to 0.38)
Divalproex sodium 250mg vs. 500mg	4 week migraine headache days: experimental phase reduction from baseline	-2.8 [2.9]	-2.2 [3.2]	-0.60 (-1.56 to 0.36)	-0.20 (-0.51 to 0.12)
Divalproex sodium 250mg vs. 500mg	Percentage of migraine headaches treated with symptomatic medications: experimental phase reduction from baseline	-7.1 [34.0]	-8.0 [29.6]	0.90 (-9.04 to 10.84)	0.03 (-0.29 to 0.34)
Divalproex sodium 250mg vs. 1000mg	Migraine headache rate: reduction from baseline, last 4 weeks	-1.7 [1.8]	-1.8 [1.8]	0.10 (-0.46 to 0.66)	0.06 (-0.26 to 0.37)
Divalproex sodium 250mg vs. 1000mg	Migraine headache rate: experimental phase % reduction from baseline	-33.1 [56.2]	-39.6 [40.4]	6.50 (-8.65 to 21.65)	0.13 (-0.18 to 0.44)
Divalproex sodium 250mg vs. 1000mg	4-week migraine headache days: experimental phase reduction from baseline	-2.8 [2.9]	-3.1 [3.6]	0.30 (-0.73 to 1.33)	0.09 (-0.22 to 0.40)
Divalproex sodium 250mg vs. 1000mg	Percentage of migraine headaches treated with symptomatic medications: experimental phase reduction from baseline	-7.1 [34.0]	-8.5 [35.9]	1.40 (-9.52 to 12.32)	0.04 (-0.27 to 0.35)
Divalproex sodium 500mg vs. 1000mg	Migraine headache rate: reduction from baseline, last 4 weeks	2.0 [1.8]	1.8 [1.8]	0.20 (-0.38 to 0.78)	0.11 (-0.21 to 0.43)
Divalproex sodium 500mg vs. 1000mg	Migraine headache rate: experimental phase % reduction from baseline	36.3 [36.9]	39.6 [40.4]	-3.30 (-15.72 to 9.12)	-0.09 (-0.41 to 0.24)
Divalproex sodium 500mg vs. 1000mg	4 week migraine headache days: experimental phase reduction from baseline	2.2 [3.2]	3.1 [3.6]	-0.90 (-1.99 to 0.19)	-0.26 (-0.59 to 0.06)
Divalproex sodium 500mg vs. 1000mg	Percentage of migraine headaches treated with symptomatic medications: experimental phase reduction from baseline	8.0 [29.6]	8.5 [35.9]	-0.50 (-11.05 to 10.05)	-0.02 (-0.34 to 0.31)

Appendix Table D42. Dose response reduction in migraine intermediate outcomes with divalproex sodium in children (results from randomized controlled clinical trials) (continued)

Compared doses	Outcome	Mean [Standard deviation] with higher dose	Mean [Standard deviation] with lower dose	Mean difference (95% CI)	Cohen standardized mean difference (95% CI)
Divalproex Sodium Extended-release 250mg vs. 500mg	Reduction from baseline: 4 week migraine headache rate	1.6 [1.7]	1.5 [1.6]	0.10 (-0.41 to 0.61)	0.06 (-0.25 to 0.37)
Divalproex Sodium Extended-release 250mg vs. 1000mg	Reduction from baseline: 4 week migraine headache rate	1.6 [1.7]	1.5 [1.6]	0.10 (-0.41 to 0.61)	0.06 (-0.25 to 0.37)
Divalproex Sodium Extended-release 500mg vs. 1000mg	Reduction from baseline: 4 week migraine headache rate	1.5 [1.6]	1.5 [1.6]	0.00 (-0.50 to 0.50)	0.00 (-0.32 to 0.32)

Appendix Table D43. Randomized controlled clinical trial that examined Internet-based self management for migraine prevention in childhood and adolescence (unclear risk of bias randomized controlled clinical trial)[18]

Reference Design Sample Number analyzed % females	Age	Definition of migraine	Presence of aura	Baseline subject characteristics	Duration of migraine	Prior treatment	Subject compliance and suitability
Trautmann, 2010[18] Design: RCT Sample: 68 Number analyzed: Not reported 54.55% females	Eligible age 10-18 years Mean age: 12.7 years	Not reported	Not reported	Headache diary: CBT: 11.5 (8.2), AR: 10.3 (7.8), Education: 10.7 (7.4), Intensity: CBT: 5.0 (1.8), AR: 5.1 (1.7), Education: 5.2 (1.70), Duration: CBT: 6.8 (4.0), AR: 8.1 (6.7), Education: 7.8 (5.8); KINDL-R: CBT: 3.6 (0.5), AR: 3.8 (0.6), Education: 3.8 (0.3); SDQ: CBT: 11.8 (3.5), AR: 8.9 (4.5), Education: 10.7 (3.9)	2.8 years	Not reported	Not reported

CBT = Multimodal cognitive-behavioral training; AR = applied relaxation; SDQ = Strength and Difficulties Questionnaire: It is a brief questionnaire with five subscales for assessing relevant psychopathological symptoms in children and adolescents. It includes 25 items with a 5-point rating scale; KINDL-R = German questionnaire that includes six dimensions of health-related quality of life)

Appendix Table D44. Migraine prevention with Internet-based self management in childhood and adolescence (unclear risk of bias randomized controlled clinical trial)[18]

Active treatment	Control treatment	Definition of the outcome	Events/randomized with active Control treatments Rate of outcome in active [control group], %	Relative risk (95% CI)	Absolute risk difference (95% CI)
Self-help training program Multimodal cognitive-behavioral training (CBT) CBT was adapted from the face-to-face group therapy program devised by Denecke and Kroener-Herwig (2000) for children with recurrent headache. CBT was reduced from 8 to 6 sessions in a self-help format, and the protocol was adapted to adolescents up to 18 years. While the first module presented education on headaches, the second unit focused on stress management (perception of own stress symptoms, coping with stress). In the following modules the participants acquired progressive relaxation techniques, cognitive restructuring (identification of dysfunctional cognitions regarding headache and stress and identifying functional cognitions), self-assurance strategies (being proactive and sensitive to one's own needs), as well as problem solving. Participants of the CBT were offered a CD with relaxation instructions (a full relaxation protocol involving tensing and relaxing of major muscle groups, beginning with the upper body and proceeding to the lower body), and they could download the relaxation instructions from the training website. The participants	Educational intervention Participants received only the first self-help module (education on headache), but they had the same number of e-mail contacts as those in the CBT and AR. The e-mails focused on the diary records of the previous week (e.g. Did you have any headache last week? What did you do?), rather than on cognitive-behavioral elements or applied relaxation instructions.	Subjective improvement of headache directly after training	12/24 9/19 50.0 [47.4]	1.1 (0.6 to 2.0)	0.03 (-0.27 to 0.33)

D-52

Appendix Table D44. Migraine prevention with Internet-based self management in childhood and adolescence (unclear risk of bias randomized controlled clinical trial) (continued)

Active treatment	Control treatment	Definition of the outcome	Events/randomized with active Control treatments Rate of outcome in active [control group], %	Relative risk (95% CI)	Absolute risk difference (95% CI)
responded to the assigned exercises and reported on their headache in the previous week through e-mail.					
Self-help training program Applied relaxation AR followed the training developed by Oˆst (1987). The self-help modules contained only several phases from the original training (Oˆst, 1987): progressive relaxation, cue-controlled relaxation and differential relaxation. Participants were offered a CD with these specific instruction tracks for the different stages of AR training to be used at home (4 tracks: a full relaxation protocol common to the CBT CD, one track of cue-controlled relaxation, two tracks for differential relaxation). The participants responded to the assigned exercises and reported on their headache in the previous week through e-mail.	Educational intervention as above.	Subjective improvement of headache directly after training	12/22 9/19 54.5 [47.4]	1.2 (0.6 to 2.1)	0.07 (-0.23 to 0.38)
Self-help training program Multimodal CBT	Applied relaxation	Subjective improvement of headache directly after training	12/24 12/22 50.0 [54.5]	0.9 (0.5 to 1.6)	-0.05 (-0.33 to 0.24)
Self-help training program Multimodal CBT	Educational intervention	Responder (50% reduction in headache frequency) at 6 weeks	10/24 2/19 41.7 [10.5]	**4.0 (1.0 to 16.0)**	**0.31 (0.07 to 0.55)**
Self-help training program Multimodal CBT	Applied relaxation	Responder (50% reduction in headache frequency) at 6 weeks	10/24 6/22 41.7 [27.3]	1.5 (0.7 to 3.5)	0.14 (-0.13 to 0.42)
Self-help training program Applied relaxation	Educational intervention	Responder (50% reduction in headache frequency) at 6 weeks	6/22 2/19 27.3 [10.5]	2.6 (0.6 to 11.4)	0.17 (-0.06 to 0.40)

Appendix Table D44. Migraine prevention with Internet-based self management in childhood and adolescence (unclear risk of bias randomized controlled clinical trial) (continued)

Active treatment	Control treatment	Definition of the outcome	Events/randomized with active Control treatments Rate of outcome in active [control group], %	Relative risk (95% CI)	Absolute risk difference (95% CI)
Self-help training program	Applied relaxation	Responder (50% reduction in headache frequency) 6 months after completion of training	9/22 5/19 40.9 [26.3]	1.6 (0.6 to 3.8)	0.15 (-0.14 to 0.43)
Self-help training program	Educational intervention	Responder (50% reduction in headache frequency) 6 months after completion of training	7/24 5/19 29.2 [26.3]	1.1 (0.4 to 2.9)	0.03 (-0.24 to 0.30)
Self-help training program	Multimodal CBT	Responder (50% reduction in headache frequency) 6 months after completion of training	7/24 9/22 29.2 [40.9]	0.7 (0.3 to 1.6)	-0.12 (-0.39 to 0.16)

CBT = Multimodal cognitive-behavioral training; AR = applied relaxation; Bold = significant at 95% confidence level when 95% CI of absolute risk difference do not include 0

Appendix Table D45. Migraine frequency with Internet-based self management for migraine prevention in childhood and adolescence (unclear risk of bias randomized controlled clinical trial)[18]

Active treatment	Control treatment	Definition of the outcome	Mean [SD] in active and control group	Mean difference (95% CI)	Standardized Cohen mean difference (95% CI)	Means ratio (95% CI)
Self-help training program Applied relaxation	Educational intervention	Headache frequency : 6 weeks	7.4 [7.60] 6.7 [6.50]	0.70 (-3.62 to 5.02)	0.10 (-0.52 to 0.71)	1.10 (0.60 to 2.04)
Self-help training program Multimodal CBT	Educational intervention	Headache duration: 6 weeks	4.8 [2.90] 6.1 [5.10]	-1.30 (-3.87 to 1.27)	-0.32 (-0.93 to 0.28)	0.79 (0.50 to 1.23)
Self-help training program Applied relaxation	Educational intervention	Headache duration: 6 weeks	6.2 [3.90] 6.1 [5.10]	0.10 (-2.71 to 2.91)	0.02 (-0.59 to 0.64)	1.02 (0.64 to 1.61)
Self-help training program Multimodal CBT	Applied relaxation	Headache frequency: 6 weeks	4.9 [4.30] 7.4 [7.60]	-2.50 (-6.11 to 1.11)	-0.41 (-0.99 to 0.18)	0.66 (0.38 to 1.15)
	Applied relaxation	Headache duration: 6 weeks	4.8 [2.90] 6.2 [3.90]	-1.40 (-3.40 to .60)	-0.41 (-0.99 to 0.17)	0.77 (0.54 to 1.11)
	Educational intervention	Headache frequency: 6 weeks	4.9 [4.30] 6.7 [6.50]	-1.80 (-5.19 to 1.59)	-0.33 (-0.94 to 0.27)	0.73 (0.42 to 1.28)
	Educational intervention	Headache intensity: 6 weeks	5.0 [2.40] 5.4 [2.00]	-0.40 (-1.72 to .92)	-0.18 (-0.78 to 0.42)	0.93 (0.72 to 1.19)
Self-help training program Applied relaxation	Educational intervention	Headache intensity: 6 weeks	5.6 [1.90] 5.4 [2.00]	0.20 (-1.00 to 1.40)	0.10 (-0.51 to 0.72)	1.04 (0.83 to 1.29)
Self-help training program Multimodal CBT	Applied relaxation	Headache intensity: 6 weeks	5.0 [2.40] 5.6 [1.90]	-0.60 (-1.85 to .65)	-0.28 (-0.86 to 0.31)	0.89 (0.70 to 1.13)

CBT = Multimodal cognitive-behavioral training; AR = applied relaxation; SD = Standard deviation

Appendix Table D46. Quality of life with Internet-based self management for migraine prevention in childhood and adolescence (unclear risk of bias randomized controlled clinical trial)[18]

Active treatment	Control treatment	Definition of the outcome	Mean [SD] in active and control group	Mean difference (95% CI)	Standardized Cohen mean difference (95% CI)	Means Ratio (95% CI)
Self-help training program Multimodal CBT	Educational intervention	Pain Catastrophisizing Scale (PCS-C) for Children: It is a self-report instrument on a 5-point rating scale: 6 weeks	27.1 [7.10] 31.7 [8.30]	-4.60 (-9.29 to 0.09)	-0.60 (-1.22 to 0.01)	0.85 (0.73 to 1.00)
Self-help training program Applied relaxation	Educational intervention	PCS-C: 6 weeks	34.7 [8.80] 31.7 [8.30]	3.00 (-2.24 to 8.24)	0.35 (-0.27 to 0.97)	1.09 (0.93 to 1.28)
Self-help training program Multimodal CBT	Educational intervention	CDI at 6 weeks (Children's Depression Inventory: German version that includes 27 items measuring cognitive, affective, and behavioral symptoms of depression in childhood on a 3-point rating scale)	11.0 [9.20] 7.7 [5.20]	3.30 (-1.06 to 7.66)	0.43 (-0.18 to 1.04)	1.43 (0.91 to 2.24)
Self-help training program Applied relaxation	Educational intervention	CDI (German version) at 6 weeks	8.1 [9.00] 7.7 [5.20]	0.40 (-4.03 to 4.83)	0.05 (-0.56 to 0.67)	1.05 (0.60 to 1.83)
Self-help training program Multimodal CBT	Educational intervention	SDQ at 6 weeks (Strength and Difficulties Questionnaire: It is a brief questionnaire with five subscales for assessing relevant psychopathological symptoms in children and adolescents. It includes 25 items with a 5-point rating scale)	11.2 [4.30] 10.0 [4.90]	1.20 (-1.60 to 4.00)	0.26 (-0.34 to 0.87)	1.12 (0.86 to 1.47)
Self-help training program Applied relaxation	Educational intervention	SDQ at 6 weeks	9.5 [4.20] 10.0 [4.90]	-0.50 (-3.32 to 2.32)	-0.11 (-0.72 to 0.50)	0.95 (0.71 to 1.27)
Self-help training program Multimodal CBT	Educational intervention	KINDL-R at 6 weeks (German KINDL - questionnaire (Ravens-	3.6 [0.40] 3.9 [0.30]	-0.30 (-0.51 to -0.09)	-0.83 (-1.46 to -0.21)	0.92 (0.87 to 0.98)

Appendix Table D46. Quality of life with Internet-based self management for migraine prevention in childhood and adolescence (unclear risk of bias randomized controlled clinical trial) (continued)

Active treatment	Control treatment	Definition of the outcome	Mean [SD] in active and control group	Mean difference (95% CI)	Standardized Cohen mean difference (95% CI)	Means Ratio (95% CI)
		Sieberer & Bullinger, 1998) that includes six dimensions of health-related quality of life)				
Self-help training program Applied relaxation	Educational intervention	German KINDL-R at 6 weeks	3.8 [0.60] 3.9 [0.30]	-0.10 (-0.38 to 0.18)	-0.21 (-0.82 to 0.41)	0.97 (0.90 to 1.05)
Self-help training program Multimodal CBT	Applied relaxation	PCS-C: 6 weeks	27.1 [7.10] 34.7 [8.80]	-7.60 (-12.25 to -2.95)	-0.96 (-1.57 to -0.34)	0.78 (0.67 to 0.91)
Self-help training program Multimodal CBT	Applied relaxation	CDI (German version) at 6 weeks	11.0 [9.20] 8.1 [9.00]	2.90 (-2.36 to 8.16)	0.32 (-0.26 to 0.90)	1.36 (0.77 to 2.41)
Self-help training program Multimodal CBT	Applied relaxation	SDQ at 6 weeks	11.2 [4.30] 9.5 [4.20]	1.70 (-0.76 to 4.16)	0.40 (-0.18 to 0.98)	1.18 (0.93 to 1.50)
Self-help training program Multimodal CBT	Applied relaxation assigned exercises and reported on their headache in the previous week through e-mail.	German KINDL-R at 6 weeks	3.6 [0.40] 3.8 [0.60]	-0.20 (-0.50 to 0.10)	-0.40 (-0.98 to 0.19)	0.95 (0.87 to 1.03)

SD = standard deviation; CBT = Multimodal cognitive-behavioral training; AR = applied relaxation; SDQ = Strength and Difficulties Questionnaire: It is a brief questionnaire with five subscales for assessing relevant psychopathological symptoms in children and adolescents. It includes 25 items with a 5-point rating scale; KINDL-R = German questionnaire that includes six dimensions of health-related quality of life); PCS-C = Pain Catastrophisizing Scale for Children: It is a self-report instrument on a 5-point rating scale

Appendix Table D47. Randomized controlled clinical trials that examined adverse effects of preventive drugs in children with migraine

Reference, Sample, Number analyzed, % female	Drug	Age	Definition of migraine	Presence of aura	Migraine duration and baseline severity	Comorbidity	Concurrent medication	Duration of migraine	Subject compliance and suitability
Battistella, 1993[4] Sample: 40 Number analyzed: Not reported 45% female	Trazodone	Eligible age 7 to 18 years Mean 12.6 years	International Headache Society criteria for migraine	All patients had migraine without aura (inclusion criterion)	History of symptoms (years), mean (SD): 4.5 (1.3); mean frequency of attacks/month: Trazodone: 4.0±0.2 and Placebo: 3.5±0.1; Mean duration of attacks in hours: Trazodone: 20.2±1.3 and Placebo: 18.2±1.1	Not reported	Not reported	4.5 years	Not reported
Wang, 2003[19] Sample: 118 Number analyzed: 118 68.6% female	Oral magnesium oxide	Eligible age Between 3 and 17 Mean 12.0 years	History of at least weekly, moderate-to-severe migraine during the previous 4 weeks and it must have been associated with anorexia/ nausea, vomiting, photophobia, sonophobia, a pulsatile or throbbing quality, or relief with sleep, but not with fever or evidence of infection.	Not reported	Headaches in last month, mean (SD) [median]: magnesium oxide: 9.3 (4.7) [8] and placebo: 11.5 (8.1) [8]	15.4% had asthma, 17% had allergies; 8.5% had depression	Patients were excluded if they took any migraine prophylactic drug therapies (such as beta-blockers, valproic acid), mg, or fever medications within 4 weeks of potential study entrance.	Age at first headache: 8.5 years	Compliance was assessed through the use of capsule counts, which were performed at week 4 and again at study's end

Appendix Table D47. Randomized controlled clinical trials that examined adverse effects of preventive drugs in children with migraine (continued)

Reference, Sample, Number analyzed, % female	Drug	Age	Definition of migraine	Presence of aura	Migraine duration and baseline severity	Comorbidity	Concurrent medication	Duration of migraine	Subject compliance and suitability
Winner, 2005[8] Sample: 162 Number analyzed: 157 48.4% female	Topiramate	Eligible age 6 to 15 years Mean 11.1 years	According to International Headache Society classification of pediatric migraine with or without aura	Not reported	Mean (SD) monthly migraine days: topiramate: 5.4 (1.7) and placebo: 5.5 (2.0)	Not reported	Not reported	Not reported	Not reported
Winner, 2006[15] Sample: 51 Number analyzed: 49 71% female	Topiramate	Eligible age 12 to 17 years Mean 14 years	International Headache Society criteria	Not reported	Migraine frequency, Mean (SD): Placebo: 4.6 (2.1), Topiramate 50mg/day: 4.8 (1.9), Topiramate 100mg/day: 6.2 (3.5), Topiramate 200mg/day: 4.9 (2.0)	Not reported	Prophylactic medications were not permitted	Not reported	Not reported
Apostol, 2008[5] U.S. Food and Drug Administration, 2008[6] Sample: 305 Number analyzed: 299 55% female	Divalproex sodium extended-release	Eligible age 12 to 17 years Mean 14.2 years	International Headache Society criteria	Not reported	Migraine headaches within 3 months prior to screening: Mean (SD): Placebo: 16.7 (7.62), 250 mg DVPX ER: 16.6 (7.02), 500 mg DVPX ER: 18.0 (7.02), 1000 mg DVPX ER:17.3 (6.84)	Not reported	Prophylactic medications were not permitted	Not reported	To document compliance with study medication, subjects were instructed to return all medication bottles and pill counts were performed. Site personnel were to counsel any subject with compliance <70%
Lewis, 2009[7] Sample: 106 Number analyzed: 103 61% female	Topiramate	Eligible age between 12 and 17 years Mean 14.2 years	International Headache Society guidelines for pediatric migraine	Not reported	Mean migraine attacks, no/month: placebo: 4.1±1.48; 50mg topiramate: 4.1±1.74 and 100mg topiramate: 4.3±1.59	Not reported	Not reported	Not reported	Subjects maintained medication records the accuracy of which was checked by their parents.

Appendix Table D47. Randomized controlled clinical trials that examined adverse effects of preventive drugs in children with migraine (continued)

Reference, Sample, Number analyzed, % female	Drug	Age	Definition of migraine	Presence of aura	Migraine duration and baseline severity	Comorbidity	Concurrent medication	Duration of migraine	Subject compliance and suitability
Pandina, 2010[17], analysis of Lewis, 2009[7] Sample: 103 Number analyzed: 103 61% female	Topiramate	Eligible age 12 to 17 years Mean: 14.2 years	International Headache Society criteria for pediatric migraine	Not reported	Not reported	Not reported	88.3% of subjects reported concomitant use of acute headache medications for migraine.	Not reported	Not reported
Sillanpää, 1977[2] Sample: 57 Number analyzed: 57 38.6% female	Clonidine	Eligible age 0-15 years Mean 11 years	Migraine was defined by the criteria of Vahlquist, i.e. paroxysmal headache separated by headache-free intervals and at least two of the following four: unilateral pain, nausea, visual aura and positive family history.	12 patients in the clonidine group and 8 in the placebo group had classic migraine with visual aura.	Frequency of headache/month (n): 5-6: Clonidine: 3 and Placebo: 4, and >6: Clonidine: 5 and Placebo: 6	Not reported	Not reported	Not reported	Not reported
Forsythe, 1984[20] Sample: 53 Number analyzed: 39 46.2% female	Propranolol	Eligible age 9 to 15 years Mean age not reported	Migraine was defined as a periodic headache with at least three of four feature: aura, nausea, vomiting, and positive family history	Not reported	Frequency of attacks: 2-5/week: Propranolol: 12 and Placebo: 4	Not reported	Not reported	Age at first attack (no.): 3-5 years: Propranolol: 3, 6-10 years: 13 and 11-12 years: 6 and Placebo: 3-5 years: 5, 6-10 years: 11 and 11-12 years: 1	As a measure of compliance, the number of tablets remaining from the dispensed was recorded

DVPX ER = Divalproex extended release; SD = standard deviation

D-60

Appendix Table D48. Adverse effects with migraine preventive drugs in children (results from nonrandomized studies)

Reference Design of study	Migraine definition Age	Drug Daily dose	Adverse effect	Events/treated Treatment weeks	Rate of outcome,%
Lewis, 2004[21] Retrospective review	International Classification of Diseases [ICD] code 884.0 and ICD codes 346.0, 346.1 and 346.2 Age <18	Amitriptyline Not reported	Discontinued treatment	2/73 Treatment weeks not reported	2.7
Apostol, 2009[22] Open-label clinical trial	International Headache Society criteria Age 12 to 17 years	Divalproex 250 to 1000mg/day	Any adverse event	203/241 Treatment weeks 48	84.2
	International Headache Society criteria Age 12 to 17 years	Divalproex 250 to 1000mg/day	Nausea	45/241 Treatment weeks 48	18.7
	International Headache Society criteria Age 12 to 17 years	Divalproex 250 to 1000mg/day	Vomiting	43/241 Treatment weeks 48	17.8
	International Headache Society criteria Age 12 to 17 years	Divalproex 250 to 1000mg/day	Weight gain	29/241 Treatment weeks 48	12.0
	International Headache Society criteria Age 12 to 17 years	Divalproex 250 to 1000mg/day	Nasopharyngitis	27/241 Treatment weeks 48	11.2
	International Headache Society criteria Age 12 to 17 years	Divalproex 250 to 1000mg/day	Migraine	25/241 Treatment weeks 48	10.4
	International Headache Society criteria Age 12 to 17 years	Divalproex 250 to 1000mg/day	Upper respiratory tract infection	25/241 Treatment weeks 48	10.4
	International Headache Society criteria Age 12 to 17 years	Divalproex 250 to 1000mg/day	One or more serious adverse effects	10/241 Treatment weeks 48	4.1
	International Headache Society criteria Age 12 to 17 years	Divalproex 250 to 1000mg/day	Irregular menses	2/241 Treatment weeks 48	0.8
Pakalnis, 2001[23] Retrospective review	International Headache Society criteria Age <17	Divalproex 250mg to 1125mg/day (3.1-32.9mg/kg/day)	Discontinued due to side effects	4/23 Treatment weeks not reported	17.4
	International Headache Society criteria Age <17	Divalproex 250mg to 1125mg/day (3.1-32.9mg/kg/day)	Discontinued due to weight gain	1/23 Treatment weeks not reported	4.3
	International Headache Society criteria Age <17	Divalproex 250mg to 1125mg/day (3.1-32.9mg/kg/day)	Discontinued due to lethargy	1/23 Treatment weeks not reported	4.3

Appendix Table D48. Adverse effects with migraine preventive drugs in children (results from nonrandomized studies) (continued)

Reference Design of study	Migraine definition Age	Drug Daily dose	Adverse effect	Events/treated Treatment weeks	Rate of outcome,%
	International Headache Society criteria Age <17	Divalproex 250mg to 1125mg/day (3.1-32.9mg/kg/day)	Discontinued due to anorexia	1/23 Treatment weeks not reported	4.3
	International Headache Society criteria Age <17	Divalproex 250mg to 1125mg/day (3.1-32.9mg/kg/day)	Discontinued due to alopecia	1/23 Treatment weeks not reported	4.3
Apostol, 2009[22] Open-label clinical trial	International Headache Society criteria Age 12 to 17 years	Divalproex 250 to 1000mg/day	Weight gain leading to discontinuation	6/241 Treatment weeks 48	2.5
	International Headache Society criteria Age 12 to 17 years	Divalproex 250 to 1000mg/day	Alopecia leading to discontinuation	5/241 Treatment weeks 48	2.1
	International Headache Society criteria Age 12 to 17 years	Divalproex 250 to 1000mg/day	Nausea leading to discontinuation	4/241 Treatment weeks 48	1.7
	International Headache Society criteria Age 12 to 17 years	Divalproex 250 to 1000mg/day	Increased ammonia leading to discontinuation	3/241 Treatment weeks 48	1.2
	International Headache Society criteria Age 12 to 17 years	Divalproex 250 to 1000mg/day	Migraine leading to discontinuation	3/241 Treatment weeks 48	1.2
	International Headache Society criteria Age 12 to 17 years	Divalproex 250 to 1000mg/day	Upper abdominal pain leading to discontinuation	2/241 Treatment weeks 48	0.8
	International Headache Society criteria Age 12 to 17 years	Divalproex 250 to 1000mg/day	Depressed mood leading to discontinuation	2/241 Treatment weeks 48	0.8
	International Headache Society criteria Age 12 to 17 years	Divalproex 250 to 1000mg/day	Depression leading to discontinuation	2/241 Treatment weeks 48	0.8
	International Headache Society criteria Age 12 to 17 years	Divalproex 250 to 1000mg/day	Irritability leading to discontinuation	2/241 Treatment weeks 48	0.8
	International Headache Society criteria Age 12 to 17 years	Divalproex 250 to 1000mg/day	Psychiatric adverse effects	4/241 Treatment weeks 48	1.7
Pakalnis, 2007[24] Prospective	ICHD-II Age 6 to 17 years	Levetiracetam 20mg/kg/day	Behavioral changes (irritability and aggressiveness)	2/22 Treatment weeks 16	9.1
	ICHD-II Age 6 to 17 years	Levetiracetam 20mg/kg/day	Mild memory problems	1/22 Treatment weeks 16	4.5

Appendix Table D48. Adverse effects with migraine preventive drugs in children (results from nonrandomized studies) (continued)

Reference Design of study	Migraine definition Age	Drug Daily dose	Adverse effect	Events/treated Treatment weeks	Rate of outcome, %
Miller, 2004[25] Retrospective review	International Headache Society criteria Age <17	Levetiracetam 125 or 250mg twice daily	Irritability and moodiness attenuated after 1 month of treatment	1/23 Treatment weeks 4	4.3
	International Headache Society criteria Age <17	Levetiracetam 125 or 250mg twice daily	Discontinued due to side effects	2/23 Treatment weeks not reported	8.7
	International Headache Society criteria Age <17	Levetiracetam 125 or 250mg twice daily	Discontinued due to asthenia/ somnolence and dizziness	1/23 Treatment weeks not reported	4.3
	International Headache Society criteria Age <17	Levetiracetam 125 or 250mg twice daily	Discontinued due to irritability, hyperactivity, and hostile behavior	1/23 Treatment weeks not reported	4.3
Cruz, 2009[26] Retrospective review	International Headache Society criteria (2004) Age <21	Topiramate 50 to 200mg/day	Cognitive decline	5/37 Treatment weeks not reported	13.5
	International Headache Society criteria (2004) Age <21	Topiramate 50 to 200mg/day	Drowsiness	3/37 Treatment weeks not reported	8.1
	International Headache Society criteria (2004) Age <21	Topiramate 50 to 200mg/day	Paresthesia	1/37 Treatment weeks not reported	2.7
	International Headache Society criteria (2004) Age <21	Topiramate 50 to 200mg/day	Anhidrosis	1/37 treatment weeks not reported	2.7
	International Headache Society criteria (2004) Age <21	Topiramate 50 to 200mg/day	Discontinued due to adverse effects	7/37 Treatment weeks not reported	18.9
	International Headache Society criteria (2004) Age <21	Topiramate 50 to 200mg/day	Discontinued due to cognitive issues	5/37 Treatment weeks not reported	13.5
	International Headache Society criteria (2004) Age <21	Topiramate 50 to 200mg/day	Discontinued due to paresthesia	1/37 Treatment weeks not reported	2.7
	International Headache Society criteria (2004) Age <21	Topiramate 50 to 200mg/day	Discontinued due to anhidrosis	1/37 t Treatment weeks not reported	2.7
Jurgens, 2011[27] Case report	Not reported Age 17 year old	Topiramate 25mg initial dose then increased gradually to 75mg/day	"Alice in Wonderland syndrome" (on 75mg/day dose and not on lower doses): Intermittent nocturnal distortions of her body image only on occasions when she did not directly fall asleep after taking topiramate.	0/1 Treatment weeks 16	

Appendix Table D48. Adverse effects with migraine preventive drugs in children (results from nonrandomized studies) (continued)

Reference Design of study	Migraine definition Age	Drug Daily dose	Adverse effect	Events/treated Treatment weeks	Rate of outcome, %
			Her head would grow bigger and the rest of the body would shrink, or that her hand resting comfortably on her chest would increase in size and become heavier, while the remaining arm would become smaller.		
Taylor, 2007[28] Retrospective and concurrent chart review	Not reported Age <18	Valproic acid Loading dose of 20-40mg/kg over one hour followed by a continuous intravenous infusion at 1-1.5mg/kg/hour	Hyperammonemia	1/26 Treatment weeks 12	3.8
	Not reported Age <18	Valproic acid Loading dose of 20-40mg/kg over one hour followed by a continuous intravenous infusion at 1-1.5mg/kg/hour	Hallucinations	1/26 Treatment weeks not reported	3.8
	Not reported Age <18	Valproic acid Loading dose of 20-40mg/kg over one hour followed by a continuous intravenous infusion at 1-1.5mg/kg/hour	Confusion (during the initial loading phase)	1/26 Treatment weeks not reported	3.8
Chan, 2009[29] Prospective	Not reported Age 14-18 years	Botox 100U every 3 months (follow-the pain approach)	Mild ptosis	1/12 Treatment weeks 12	8.3
	Not reported Age 14-18 years	Botox 100U every 3 months (follow-the pain approach)	Blurred vision	1/12 Treatment weeks 12	8.3
	Not reported Age 14-18 years	Botox 100U every 3 months (follow-the pain approach)	Hematoma at one of neck injection site with resultant tingling in one arm lasting 24 hours	1/12 Treatment weeks not reported	8.3
	Not reported Age 14-18 years	Botox 100U every 3 months (follow-the pain approach)	Burning sensations at all injection sites lasting 1 week	1/12 Treatment weeks 116	8.3

ICHD II = International Headache Society, second edition

D-64

Appendix Table D49. Treatment discontinuation due to adverse effects with topiramate for migraine prevention in children (pooled with random effects model results from randomized controlled clinical trials)

Outcome	Dose	Reference, Risk of bias	Events/ Randomized [rate, %] with drug	Events/ Randomized [rate, %] with placebo	Relative risk (95% CI)	Weight	Absolute risk difference (95% CI)	Weight
Treatment discontinuation	50mg	Lewis, 2009[7] Low	6/35 [17.1]	7/33 [21.2]	0.8 (0.3 to 2.2)	17.56	-0.04(-0.23 to 0.15)	19.67
Treatment discontinuation	50mg	Winner, 2006[15] Low	4/12 [33.3]	5/12 [41.7]	0.8 (0.3 to 2.3)	15.53	-0.08(-0.47 to 0.30)	4.63
Treatment discontinuation	50mg	Pooled	10/47 [21.3]	12/45 [26.7]	0.8 (0.4 to 1.6)	33.09	-0.05(-0.22 to 0.12)	24.29
Treatment discontinuation	100mg	Lewis, 2009[7] Low	5/35 [14.3]	7/33 [21.2]	0.8 (0.4 to 1.6)	15.5	-0.05(-0.22 to 0.12)	20.95
Treatment discontinuation	100mg	Winner, 2006[15] Low	3/13 [23.1]	5/12 [41.7]	0.7 (0.2 to 1.9)	11.8	-0.07(-0.25 to 0.11)	5.29
Treatment discontinuation	100mg	Pooled	8/48 [16.7]	12/45 [26.7]	0.6 (0.2 to 1.8)	27.3	-0.19(-0.55 to 0.18)	26.24
Treatment discontinuation	200mg	Winner, 2006[15] Low	2/14 [14.3]	5/12 [41.7]	0.3 (0.1 to 1.5)	8.07	-0.27(-0.61 to 0.06)	6.19
Treatment discontinuation	200mg	Winner, 2005[8] Medium	23/112 [20.5]	8/50 [16.0]	1.3 (0.6 to 2.7)	31.54	0.05(-0.08 to 0.17)	43.28
Treatment discontinuation	200mg	Pooled	25/126 [19.8]	13/62 [21.0]	0.8 (0.2 to 2.7)	39.61	-0.08(-0.38 to 0.23)	49.47
Treatment discontinuation	Overall	Pooled	55/281 [19.6]	54/209 [25.8]	0.8 (0.5 to 1.2)	100	-0.03(-0.12 to 0.05)	100
Treatment discontinuation	Heterogeneity	Degree of freedom	Groups	P	I-squared	Groups	P	I-squared
Treatment discontinuation	50mg	1	50mg	0.989	0.00%	50mg	0.846	0.00%
Treatment discontinuation	100mg	1	100mg	0.809	0.00%	100mg	0.571	0.00%
Treatment discontinuation	200mg	1	200mg	0.111	60.70%	200mg	0.08	67.50%
Treatment discontinuation	Overall	5	Overall	0.641	0.00%	Overall	0.494	0.00%
Treatment discontinuation due to adverse events	50mg	Lewis, 2009[7] Low	3/35 [8.6]	1/33 [3.0]	2.8 (0.3 to 25.9)	24.53	0.06(-0.05 to 0.17)	22.6
Treatment	100mg	Lewis, 2009[7]	3/35	1/33	2.8 (0.3 to 25.9)	24.53	0.06(-0.05 to 0.17)	22.6

Appendix Table D49. Treatment discontinuation due to adverse effects with topiramate for migraine prevention in children (pooled with random effects model results from randomized controlled clinical trials) (continued)

Outcome	Dose	Reference, Risk of bias	Events/ Randomized [rate, %] with drug	Events/ Randomized [rate, %] with placebo	Relative risk (95% CI)	Weight	Absolute risk difference (95% CI)	Weight
discontinuation due to adverse events		Low	[8.6]	[3.0]				
Treatment discontinuation due to adverse events	200mg	Winner, 2005[8] Medium	7/112 [6.3]	2/50 [4.0]	1.6 (0.3 to 7.3)	50.93	0.02(-0.05 to 0.09)	54.79
Treatment discontinuation due to adverse events	Pooled		13/182 [7.1]	4/116 [3.4]	2.1 (0.7 to 6.3)	100	0.04(-0.02 to 0.09)	100
Treatment discontinuation due to adverse events	Heterogeneity	Degree of freedom	Groups	P	I-squared	Groups	P	I-squared
Treatment discontinuation due to adverse events	Overall	2	Overall	0.869	0.00%	Overall	0.827	0.00%

Appendix Table D50. Strength of evidence about treatment discontinuation due to adverse effects with antiepileptic drugs for migraine prevention in children

Active drug	Dose	Rate with drug, % [placebo]	RCTs	Children	Directness	Risk of bias	Consistency	Precision	Dose response	Strength of evidence	Conclusion
Divalproex sodium U.S. Food and Drug Administration[6] Apostol, 2008[5]	1000mg	9.3 [1.4]	1	148	Yes	Low	Yes	No	Yes	Low	Divalproex sodium 1000mg resulted in greater treatment discontinuation rates vs. placebo
	250mg	2.4 [1.4]	1	156	Yes	Low	Yes	No	Yes	Low	Divalproex sodium 250mg did not result in greater treatment discontinuation rates vs. placebo
Topiramate Lewis, 2009[7] Pandina, 2010[17], Winner, 2005[8]	50-200mg	7.1[3.4]	2	265	Yes	Medium	Yes	No	No	Low	Topiramate did not result in greater treatment discontinuation rates vs. placebo

Appendix Table D51. Adverse effects with topiramate vs. placebo in children (results from randomized controlled clinical trials)

Outcome	Reference Risk of bias	Dose	Events/randomized [rate, %] with drug	Events/randomized [rate, %] with placebo	Relative risk (95% CI)	Absolute risk difference (95% CI)
Abnormal vision	Lewis, 2009[7]* Low	50mg	1/35 [2.9]	1/33 [3.0]	0.9 (0.1 to 14.5)	0.00 (-0.08 to 0.08)
	Lewis, 2009[7] Low	100mg	2/35 [5.7]	1/33 [3.0]	1.9 (0.2 to 19.8)	0.03 (-0.07 to 0.12)
Allergy	Lewis, 2009[7] Low	100mg	2/35 [5.7]	0/33 [0.0]	4.7 (0.2 to 94.8)	0.06 (-0.04 to 0.15)
Any adverse event	Winner, 2006[15] Low	100mg	11/13 [84.6]	10/12 [83.3]	1.0 (0.7 to 1.4)	0.01 (-0.28 to 0.30)
	Winner, 2006[15] Risk of bias Low	200mg	12/14 [85.7]	10/12 [83.3]	1.0 (0.7 to 1.4)	0.02 (-0.26 to 0.30)
	Winner, 2006[15] Low	50mg	8/12 [66.7]	10/12 [83.3]	0.8 (0.5 to 1.3)	-0.17 (-0.51 to 0.17)
Any treatment related adverse event	**Lewis, 2009[7] Low**	**50mg**	**26/35 [74.3]**	**16/33 [48.5]**	**1.5 (1.0 to 2.3)**	**0.26 (0.03 to 0.48)**
	Lewis, 2009[7] Low	**100mg**	**26/35 [74.3]**	**16/33 [48.5]**	**1.5 (1.0 to 2.3)**	**0.26 (0.03 to 0.48)**
Asthma	Lewis, 2009[7] Low	100mg	2/35 [5.7]	0/33 [0.0]	4.7 (0.2 to 94.8)	0.06 (-0.04 to 0.15)
Back pain	Lewis, 2009[7] Low	50mg	0/35 [0.0]	3/33 [9.1]	0.1 (0.0 to 2.5)	-0.09 (-0.20 to 0.02)
	Lewis, 2009[7] Low	100mg	2/35 [5.7]	3/33 [9.1]	0.6 (0.1 to 3.5)	-0.03 (-0.16 to 0.09)
Bronchitis	Winner, 2006[15] Low	100mg	1/13 [7.7]	1/12 [8.3]	0.9 (0.1 to 13.2)	-0.01 (-0.22 to 0.21)
	Winner, 2006[15] Low	200mg	0/14 [0.0]	1/12 [8.3]	0.3 (0.0 to 6.5)	-0.08 (-0.28 to 0.11)
	Winner, 2006[15] Risk of bias Low	50mg	0/12 [0.0]	1/12 [8.3]	0.3 (0.0 to 7.5)	-0.08 (-0.29 to 0.12)
Conjunctivitis	Lewis, 2009[7] Low	50mg	3/35 [8.6]	1/33 [3.0]	2.8 (0.3 to 25.9)	0.06 (-0.05 to 0.17)
	Lewis, 2009[7] Low	100mg	1/35 [2.9]	1/33 [3.0]	0.9 (0.1 to 14.5)	0.00 (-0.08 to 0.08)
Cough	Lewis, 2009[7] Risk of bias Low	50mg	3/35 [8.6]	0/33 [0.0]	6.6 (0.4 to 123.3)	0.09 (-0.02 to 0.19)
	Lewis, 2009[7] Low	100mg	1/35 [2.9]	0/33 [0.0]	2.8 (0.1 to 67.2)	0.03 (-0.05 to 0.11)
Depression	Pandina, 2010[17] Low	50mg	1/35 [2.9]	0/33 [0.0]	2.8 (0.1 to 67.2)	0.03 (-0.05 to 0.11)

Appendix Table D51. Adverse effects with topiramate vs. placebo in children (results from randomized controlled clinical trials) (continued)

Outcome	Reference Risk of bias	Dose	Events/randomized [rate, %] with drug	Events/randomized [rate, %] with placebo	Relative risk (95% CI)	Absolute risk difference (95% CI)
Diarrhea	Winner, 2006[15] Low	100mg	1/13 [7.7]	0/12 [0.0]	2.8 (0.1 to 62.5)	0.08 (-0.12 to 0.27)
	Winner, 2006[15] Low	200mg	1/14 [7.1]	0/12 [0.0]	2.6 (0.1 to 58.5)	0.07 (-0.11 to 0.26)
Difficulty concentration/attention	Pandina, 2010[17] Low	100mg	1/35 [2.9]	0/33 [0.0]	2.8 (0.1 to 67.2)	0.03 (-0.05 to 0.11)
	Winner, 2006[15] Low	200mg	2/14 [14.3]	0/12 [0.0]	4.3 (0.2 to 82.3)	0.14 (-0.07 to 0.36)
Difficulty memory numbers	Winner, 2006[15] Low	100mg	0/13 [0.0]	1/12 [8.3]	0.3 (0.0 to 6.9)	-0.08 (-0.28 to 0.12)
	Winner, 2006[15] Low	200mg	1/14 [7.1]	1/12 [8.3]	0.9 (0.1 to 12.3)	-0.01 (-0.22 to 0.19)
	Winner, 2006[15] Low	50mg	0/12 [0.0]	1/12 [8.3]	0.3 (0.0 to 7.5)	-0.08 (-0.29 to 0.12)
Emotional stress	Pandina, 2010[17] Low	50mg	1/35 [2.9]	0/33 [0.0]	2.8 (0.1 to 67.2)	0.03 (-0.05 to 0.11)
Eye pain	Lewis, 2009[7] Low	50mg	1/35 [2.9]	2/33 [6.1]	0.5 (0.0 to 5.0)	-0.03 (-0.13 to 0.07)
	Lewis, 2009[7] Low	100mg	1/35 [2.9]	2/33 [6.1]	0.5 (0.0 to 5.0)	-0.03 (-0.13 to 0.07)
Fever	Lewis, 2009[7] Low	50mg	2/35 [5.7]	0/33 [0.0]	4.7 (0.2 to 94.8)	0.06 (-0.04 to 0.15)
	Winner, 2005[8] Medium	200mg	6/112 [5.4]	2/50 [4.0]	1.3 (0.3 to 6.4)	0.01 (-0.05 to 0.08)
	Lewis, 2009[7] Low	100mg	2/35 [5.7]	0/33 [0.0]	4.7 (0.2 to 94.8)	0.06 (-0.04 to 0.15)
Gastroenteritis	Winner, 2005[8] Medium	200mg	10/112 [8.9]	3/50 [6.0]	1.5 (0.4 to 5.2)	0.03 (-0.06 to 0.11)
Infection, viral	Winner, 2006[15] Low	100mg	1/13 [7.7]	1/12 [8.3]	0.9 (0.1 to 13.2)	-0.01 (-0.22 to 0.21)
	Winner, 2006[15] Low	200mg	2/14 [14.3]	1/12 [8.3]	1.7 (0.2 to 16.6)	0.06 (-0.18 to 0.30)
	Winner, 2006[15] Low	50mg	1/12 [8.3]	1/12 [8.3]	1.0 (0.1 to 14.2)	0.00 (-0.22 to 0.22)
Influenza-like symptoms	Winner, 2005[8] Medium	200mg	8/112 [7.1]	2/50 [4.0]	1.8 (0.4 to 8.1)	0.03 (-0.04 to 0.10)
Language problems	Winner, 2006[15] Low	100mg	0/13 [0.0]	1/12 [8.3]	0.3 (0.0 to 6.9)	-0.08 (-0.28 to 0.12)
	Winner, 2006[15]	200mg	2/14		1.7 (0.2 to 16.6)	0.06 (-0.18 to 0.30)

Appendix Table D51. Adverse effects with topiramate vs. placebo in children (results from randomized controlled clinical trials) (continued)

Outcome	Reference Risk of bias	Dose	Events/randomized [rate, %] with drug	Events/randomized [rate, %] with placebo	Relative risk (95% CI)	Absolute risk difference (95% CI)
	Low		[14.3]	[8.3]		
	Winner, 2006[15] Low	50mg	0/12 [0.0]	1/12 [8.3]	0.3 (0.0 to 7.5)	-0.08 (-0.29 to 0.12)
Pneumonia	Lewis, 2009[7] Low	100mg	2/35 [5.7]	0/33 [0.0]	4.7 (0.2 to 94.8)	0.06 (-0.04 to 0.15)
Psychomotor slowing	Winner, 2006[15] Low	200mg	1/14 [7.1]	0/12 [0.0]	2.6 (0.1 to 58.5)	0.07 (-0.11 to 0.26)
	Winner, 2006[15] Low	50mg	1/12 [8.3]	0/12 [0.0]	3.0 (0.1 to 67.1)	0.08 (-0.12 to 0.29)
Taste perversion	Lewis, 2009[7] Low	50mg	1/35 [2.9]	0/33 [0.0]	2.8 (0.1 to 67.2)	0.03 (-0.05 to 0.11)
	Lewis, 2009[7] Low	100mg	3/35 [8.6]	0/33 [0.0]	6.6 (0.4 to 123.3)	0.09 (-0.02 to 0.19)
Viral infection	Lewis, 2009[7] Low	50mg	1/35 [2.9]	1/33 [3.0]	0.9 (0.1 to 14.5)	0.00 (-0.08 to 0.08)
	Lewis, 2009[7] Low	100mg	3/35 [8.6]	1/33 [3.0]	2.8 (0.3 to 25.9)	0.06 (-0.05 to 0.17)
Vomiting	Lewis, 2009[7] Low	50mg	0/35 [0.0]	1/33 [3.0]	0.3 (0.0 to 7.5)	-0.03 (-0.11 to 0.05)
	Lewis, 2009[7] Low	100mg	2/35 [5.7]	1/33 [3.0]	1.9 (0.2 to 19.8)	0.03 (-0.07 to 0.12)

Bold = significant differences when 95% CI of absolute risk difference do not include 0, * = at the investigator's discretion the dose was increased to the maximal dose tolerated by the subjects, 91% achieved the target daily dose during the double-blind treatment phase, the daily dose used during the entire double-blind treatment phase (titration and maintenance) was 73.6 ±18.7 mg/day

D-70

Appendix Table D52. Adverse effects with topiramate vs. placebo in children (pooled with random effects results from randomized controlled clinical trials)

Outcome	Dose	Reference, Risk of bias	Events/Randomized [rate, %] with drug	Events/Randomized [rate, %] with placebo	Relative risk (95% CI)	Weight	Absolute risk difference (95% CI)	Weight
Abdominal pain	50mg	Lewis, 2009[7] Low	3/35 [8.6]	3/33 [9.1]	0.9(0.2 to 4.3)	16.43	-0.01(-0.14 to 0.13)	22.37
Abdominal pain	50mg	Winner, 2006[15] Low	0/12 [0.0]	1/12 [8.3]	0.3(0.0 to 7.5)	3.97	-0.08(-0.29 to 0.12)	9.92
Abdominal pain		Pooled	3/47 [6.4]	4/45 [8.9]	0.8(0.2 to 3.0)	20.4	-0.03(-0.14 to 0.08)	32.28
Abdominal pain	100mg	Lewis, 2009[7] Low	5/35 [14.3]	3/33 [9.1]	1.6(0.4 to 6.1)	21.05	0.05(-0.10 to 0.20)	17.67
Abdominal pain	100mg	Winner, 2006[15] Low	2/13 [15.4]	1/12 [8.3]	1.8(0.2 to 17.8)	7.45	0.07(-0.18 to 0.32)	6.48
Abdominal pain		Pooled	7/48 [14.6]	4/45 [8.9]	1.6(0.5 to 5.2)	28.5	0.06(-0.07 to 0.19)	24.15
Abdominal pain	200mg	Winner, 2005[8] Medium	11/112 [9.8]	6/50 [12.0]	0.8(0.3 to 2.1)	43.67	-0.02(-0.13 to 0.08)	36.55
Abdominal pain	200mg	Winner, 2006[15] Low	2/14 [14.3]	1/12 [8.3]	1.7(0.2 to 16.6)	7.42	0.06(-0.18 to 0.30)	7.02
Abdominal pain		Pooled	13/126 [10.3]	7/62 [11.3]	0.9(0.4 to 2.2)	51.1	-0.01(-0.11 to 0.09)	43.57
Abdominal pain		Pooled	23/221 [10.4]	15/152 [9.9]	1.0(0.6 to 1.9)	100	0.00(-0.06 to 0.06)	100
Anorexia	50mg	Lewis, 2009[7] Low	3/35 [8.6]	1/33 [3.0]	2.8(0.3 to 25.9)	11.32	0.06(-0.05 to 0.17)	26.37
Anorexia	50mg	Winner, 2006[15] Low	1/12 [8.3]	1/12 [8.3]	1.0(0.1 to 14.2)	7.87	0.00(-0.22 to 0.22)	6.48
Anorexia		Pooled	4/47 [8.5]	2/45 [4.4]	1.8(0.3 to 10.1)	19.19	0.04(-0.05 to 0.14)	32.85
Anorexia	100mg	Lewis, 2009[7] Low	4/35 [11.4]	1/33 [3.0]	3.8(0.4 to 32.0)	12.11	0.08(-0.04 to 0.21)	21.81
Anorexia	100mg	Winner, 2006[15] Low	1/13 [7.7]	1/12 [8.3]	0.9(0.1 to 13.2)	7.84	-0.01(-0.22 to 0.21)	6.98
Anorexia		Pooled	5/48 [10.4]	2/45 [4.4]	2.2(0.4 to 11.5)	19.95	0.06(-0.04 to 0.17)	28.79
Anorexia	200mg	Winner, 2005[8] Medium	15/112 [13.4]	4/50 [8.0]	1.7(0.6 to 4.8)	50.14	0.05(-0.04 to 0.15)	32.9
Anorexia	200mg	Winner, 2006[15] Low	2/14 [14.3]	1/12 [8.3]	1.7(0.2 to 16.6)	10.72	0.06(-0.18 to 0.30)	5.46
Anorexia		Pooled	17/126	5/62	1.7(0.6 to 4.4)	60.86	0.06(-0.04 to 0.15)	38.36

Appendix Table D52. Adverse effects with topiramate vs. placebo in children (pooled with random effects results from randomized controlled clinical trials) (continued)

Outcome	Dose	Reference, Risk of bias	Events/ Randomized [rate, %] with drug	Events/ Randomized [rate, %] with placebo	Relative risk (95% CI)	Weight	Absolute risk difference (95% CI)	Weight
Anorexia		Pooled	26/221 [11.8]	9/152 [5.9]	1.8(0.9 to 3.8)	100	0.05(0.00 to 0.11)	100
Dizziness	50mg	Lewis, 2009[7] Low	2/35 [5.7]	0/33 [0.0]	4.7(0.2 to 94.8)	19.56	0.06(-0.04 to 0.15)	30.22
Dizziness	50mg	Winner, 2006[15] Low	0/12 [0.0]	2/12 [16.7]	0.2(0.0 to 3.8)	20.11	-0.17(-0.41 to 0.07)	13.56
Dizziness		Pooled	2/47 [4.3]	2/45 [4.4]	1.0(0.0 to 21.2)	39.67	-0.03(-0.24 to 0.19)	43.78
Dizziness	100mg	Lewis, 2009[7] Low	3/35 [8.6]	0/353 [0.0]	6.6(0.4 to 123.3)	20.21	0.09(-0.02 to 0.19)	28.43
Dizziness	100mg	Winner, 2006[15] Low	0/13 [0.0]	2/12 [16.7]	0.2(0.0 to 3.5)	20.07	-0.17(-0.40 to 0.07)	13.79
Dizziness		Pooled	3/48 [6.3]	2/365 [4.4]	1.1(0.0 to 36.8)	40.28	-0.02(-0.26 to 0.23)	42.23
Dizziness	200mg	Winner, 2006[15] Low	0/14 [0.0]	2/12 [16.7]	0.2(0.0 to 3.3)	20.05	-0.17(-0.40 to 0.07)	13.99
Dizziness		Pooled	5/109 [4.6]	6/422 [5.9]	0.7(0.1 to 3.7)	100	-0.03(-0.14 to 0.08)	100
Fatigue	50mg	Lewis, 2009[7] Low	2/35 [5.7]	2/33 [6.1]	0.9(0.1 to 6.3)	13.98	0.00(-0.12 to 0.11)	25.91
Fatigue	50mg	Winner, 2006[15] Low	0/12 [0.0]	1/12 [8.3]	0.3(0.0 to 7.5)	5.23	-0.08(-0.29 to 0.12)	7.91
Fatigue		Pooled	2/47 [4.3]	3/45 [6.7]	0.7(0.1 to 3.6)	19.21	-0.02(-0.12 to 0.08)	33.82
Fatigue	100mg	Lewis, 2009[7] Low	3/35 [8.6]	2/33 [6.1]	1.4(0.3 to 7.9)	16.98	0.03(-0.10 to 0.15)	21.34
Fatigue	100mg	Winner, 2006[15] Low	1/13 [7.7]	1/12 [8.3]	0.9(0.1 to 13.2)	7.15	-0.01(-0.22 to 0.21)	7.15
Fatigue		Pooled	4/48 [8.3]	3/45 [6.7]	1.2(0.3 to 5.3)	24.13	0.02(-0.09 to 0.12)	28.49
Fatigue	200mg	Winner, 2005[8] Medium	7/112 [6.3]	6/50 [12.0]	0.5(0.2 to 1.5)	46.88	-0.06(-0.16 to 0.04)	32.1
Fatigue	200mg	Winner, 2006[15] Low	2/14 [14.3]	1/12 [8.3]	1.7(0.2 to 16.6)	9.78	0.06(-0.18 to 0.30)	5.6
Fatigue		Pooled	9/126 [7.1]	7/62 [11.3]	0.6(0.2 to 1.6)	56.66	-0.04(-0.13 to 0.05)	37.7
Fatigue		Pooled	15/221	13/152	0.8(0.4 to 1.6)	100	-0.02(-0.08 to 0.04)	100

Appendix Table D52. Adverse effects with topiramate vs. placebo in children (pooled with random effects results from randomized controlled clinical trials) (continued)

Outcome	Dose	Reference, Risk of bias	Events/ Randomized [rate, %] with drug	Events/ Randomized [rate, %] with placebo	Relative risk (95% CI)	Weight	Absolute risk difference (95% CI)	Weight
			[6.8]	[8.6]				
Injury	50mg	Lewis, 2009[7] Low	3/35 [8.6]	2/33 [6.1]	1.4(0.3 to 7.9)	15.79	0.03(-0.10 to 0.15)	23.1
Injury	50mg	Winner, 2006[15] Low	1/12 [8.3]	1/12 [8.3]	1.0(0.1 to 14.2)	6.67	0.00(-0.22 to 0.22)	7.19
Injury		Pooled	4/47 [8.5]	3/45 [6.7]	1.3(0.3 to 5.4)	22.47	0.02(-0.09 to 0.13)	30.3
Injury	100mg	Lewis, 2009[7] Low	4/35 [11.4]	2/33 [6.1]	1.9(0.4 to 9.6)	17.7	0.05(-0.08 to 0.19)	19.84
Injury	100mg	Winner, 2006[15] Low	1/13 [7.7]	1/12 [8.3]	0.9(0.1 to 13.2)	6.65	-0.01(-0.22 to 0.21)	7.74
Injury		Pooled	5/48 [10.4]	3/45 [6.7]	1.6(0.4 to 6.2)	24.35	0.04(-0.08 to 0.15)	27.58
Injury	200mg	Winner, 2005[8] Medium	8/112 [7.1]	6/50 [12.0]	0.6(0.2 to 1.6)	46.56	-0.05(-0.15 to 0.05)	33.87
Injury	200mg	Winner, 2006[15] Low	1/14 [7.1]	1/12 [8.3]	0.9(0.1 to 12.3)	6.63	-0.01(-0.22 to 0.20)	8.25
Injury		Pooled	9/126 [7.1]	7/62 [11.3]	0.6(0.2 to 1.6)	53.19	-0.04(-0.13 to 0.05)	42.12
Injury		Pooled	18/221 [8.1]	13/152 [8.6]	0.9(0.5 to 1.8)	100	0.00(-0.06 to 0.06)	100
Mood problems	50mg	Winner, 2006[15] Low	0/12 [0.0]	2/12 [16.7]	0.2(0.0 to 3.8)	18.56	-0.17(-0.41 to 0.07)	7.29
Mood problems	50mg	20159428 Low	1/35 [2.9]	0/33 [0.0]	2.8(0.1 to 67.2)	15.97	0.03(-0.05 to 0.11)	39.29
Mood problems		Pooled	1/47 [2.1]	2/45 [4.4]	0.7(0.1 to 9.4)	34.53	-0.04(-0.21 to 0.14)	46.58
Mood problems	100mg	Winner, 2006[15] Low	0/13 [0.0]	2/12 [16.7]	0.2(0.0 to 3.5)	18.51	-0.17(-0.40 to 0.07)	7.47
Mood problems	100mg	20159428 Low	1/35 [2.9]	0/33 [0.0]	2.8(0.1 to 67.2)	15.97	0.03(-0.05 to 0.11)	39.29
Mood problems		Pooled	1/48 [2.1]	2/45 [4.4]	0.7(0.0 to 9.8)	34.48	-0.04(-0.22 to 0.14)	46.75
Mood problems	200mg	Winner, 2006[15] Low	1/14 [7.1]	2/12 [16.7]	0.4(0.0 to 4.2)	30.98	-0.10(-0.35 to 0.16)	6.67
Mood problems		Pooled	3/109 [2.8]	6/102 [5.9]	0.6(0.2 to 2.1)	100	-0.01(-0.08 to 0.06)	100
Nausea	50mg	Lewis, 2009[7]	2/35	2/33	0.9(0.1 to 6.3)	23.74	0.00(-0.12 to 0.11)	25.71

Appendix Table D52. Adverse effects with topiramate vs. placebo in children (pooled with random effects results from randomized controlled clinical trials) (continued)

Outcome	Dose	Reference, Risk of bias	Events/ Randomized [rate, %] with drug	Events/ Randomized [rate, %] with placebo	Relative risk (95% CI)	Weight	Absolute risk difference (95% CI)	Weight
Nausea	100mg	Lewis, 2009[7] Low	[5.7] 3/35 [8.6]	[6.1] 2/33 [6.1]	1.4(0.3 to 7.9)	28.84	0.03(-0.10 to 0.15)	21.18
Nausea	200mg	Winner, 2005[8] Medium	6/112 [5.4]	3/50 [6.0]	0.9(0.2 to 3.4)	47.42	-0.01(-0.08 to 0.07)	53.11
Nausea		Pooled	11/182 [6.0]	7/116 [6.0]	1.0(0.4 to 2.6)	100	0.00(-0.06 to 0.06)	100
Paresthesia	50mg	Lewis, 2009[7] Low	8/35 [22.9]	1/33 [3.0]	7.5(1.0 to 57.1)	14.01	0.20(0.05 to 0.35)	9.89
Paresthesia	50mg	Winner, 2006[15] Low	1/12 [8.3]	2/12 [16.7]	0.5(0.1 to 4.8)	11.2	-0.08(-0.35 to 0.18)	3.27
Paresthesia		Pooled	9/47 [19.1]	3/45 [6.7]	2.0(0.1 to 29.1)	25.21	0.08(-0.19 to 0.35)	13.16
Paresthesia	100mg	Lewis, 2009[7] Low	4/35 [11.4]	1/33 [3.0]	3.8(0.4 to 32.0)	12.54	0.08(-0.04 to 0.21)	15.5
Paresthesia	100mg	Winner, 2006[15] Low	5/13 [38.5]	2/12 [16.7]	2.3(0.5 to 9.7)	27.67	0.22(-0.12 to 0.56)	1.97
Paresthesia		Pooled	9/48 [18.8]	3/45 [6.7]	2.7(0.8 to 8.9)	40.21	0.10(-0.01 to 0.21)	17.47
Paresthesia	200mg	Winner, 2005[8] Medium	9/112 [8.0]	0/50 [0.0]	8.6(0.5 to 144.5)	7.19	0.08(0.02 to 0.14)	67.27
Paresthesia	200mg	Winner, 2006[15] Low	5/14 [35.7]	2/12 [16.7]	2.1(0.5 to 9.1)	27.39	0.19(-0.14 to 0.52)	2.1
Paresthesia		Pooled	14/126 [11.1]	2/62 [3.2]	2.9(0.8 to 10.4)	34.58	0.08(0.03 to 0.14)	69.37
Paresthesia		**Pooled**	**32/221 [14.5]**	**8/152 [5.3]**	**2.6(1.2 to 5.6)**	**100**	**0.09(0.05 to 0.14)**	**100**
Sinusitis	50mg	Lewis, 2009[7] Low	2/35 [5.7]	1/33 [3.0]	1.9(0.2 to 19.8)	10.17	0.03(-0.07 to 0.12)	25.26
Sinusitis	50mg	Winner, 2006[15] Low	1/12 [8.3]	0/12 [0.0]	3.0(0.1 to 67.1)	5.83	0.08(-0.12 to 0.29)	5.74
Sinusitis		Pooled	3/47 [6.4]	1/45 [2.2]	2.2(0.3 to 14.6)	16.01	0.04(-0.05 to 0.13)	30.99
Sinusitis	100mg	Lewis, 2009[7] Low	1/35 [2.9]	1/33 [3.0]	0.9(0.1 to 14.5)	7.55	0.00(-0.08 to 0.08)	36.45
Sinusitis	100mg	Winner, 2006[15] Low	1/13 [7.7]	0/12 [0.0]	2.8(0.1 to 62.5)	5.82	0.08(-0.12 to 0.27)	6.34
Sinusitis		Pooled	2/48	1/45	1.5(0.2 to 11.8)	13.37	0.01(-0.06 to 0.08)	42.8

Appendix Table D52. Adverse effects with topiramate vs. placebo in children (pooled with random effects results from randomized controlled clinical trials) (continued)

Outcome	Dose	Reference, Risk of bias	Events/ Randomized [rate, %] with drug	Events/ Randomized [rate, %] with placebo	Relative risk (95% CI)	Weight	Absolute risk difference (95% CI)	Weight
Sinusitis	200mg	Winner, 2005[8] Medium	11/112 [9.8]	6/50 [12.0]	0.8(0.3 to 2.1)	64.12	-0.02(-0.13 to 0.08)	21.14
Sinusitis	200mg	Winner, 2006[15] Low	2/14 [14.3]	0/12 [0.0]	4.3(0.2 to 82.3)	6.5	0.14(-0.07 to 0.36)	5.07
Sinusitis		Pooled	13/126 [10.3]	6/62 [9.7]	1.0(0.3 to 3.1)	70.62	0.03(-0.12 to 0.18)	26.21
Sinusitis		Pooled	18/221 [8.1]	8/152 [5.3]	1.2(0.5 to 2.5)	100	0.02(-0.03 to 0.07)	100
Somnolence	50mg	Winner, 2006[15] Low	1/12 [8.3]	1/12 [8.3]	1.0(0.1 to 14.2)	11.69	0.00(-0.22 to 0.22)	6.34
Somnolence	100mg	Lewis, 2009[7] Low	2/35 [5.7]	0/33 [0.0]	4.7(0.2 to 94.8)	9.15	0.06(-0.04 to 0.15)	36.34
Somnolence	100mg	Winner, 2006[15] Low	1/13 [7.7]	1/12 [8.3]	0.9(0.1 to 13.2)	11.65	-0.01(-0.22 to 0.21)	6.82
Somnolence		Pooled	3/48 [6.3]	1/45 [2.2]	1.9(0.3 to 13.8)	20.8	0.05(-0.04 to 0.13)	43.17
Somnolence	200mg	Winner, 2005[8] Medium	9/112 [8.0]	3/50 [6.0]	1.3(0.4 to 4.7)	51.58	0.02(-0.06 to 0.10)	45.15
Somnolence	200mg	Winner, 2006[15] Low	2/14 [14.3]	1/12 [8.3]	1.7(0.2 to 16.6)	15.93	0.06(-0.18 to 0.30)	5.34
Somnolence		Pooled	11/126 [8.7]	4/62 [6.5]	1.4(0.5 to 4.3)	67.51	0.03(-0.05 to 0.10)	50.49
Somnolence		Pooled	15/186 [8.1]	6/119 [5.0]	1.4(0.6 to 3.6)	100	0.03(-0.02 to 0.09)	100
Upper respiratory tract infection	50mg	Lewis, 2009[7] Low	7/35 [20.0]	3/33 [9.1]	2.2(0.6 to 7.8)	16.37	0.11(-0.06 to 0.27)	21.42
Upper respiratory tract infection	50mg	Winner, 2006[15] Low	5/12 [41.7]	1/12 [8.3]	5.0(0.7 to 36.7)	6.61	0.33(0.01 to 0.65)	5.69
Upper respiratory tract infection		Pooled	12/47 [25.5]	4/45 [8.9]	2.8(1.0 to 8.1)	22.99	0.18(-0.03 to 0.38)	27.11
Upper respiratory tract infection	100mg	Lewis, 2009[7] Low	8/35 [22.9]	3/33 [9.1]	2.5(0.7 to 8.7)	17.11	0.14(-0.03 to 0.31)	20.09
Upper respiratory tract infection	100mg	Winner, 2006[15] Low	3/13 [23.1]	1/12 [8.3]	2.8(0.3 to 23.1)	5.83	0.15(-0.13 to 0.43)	7.57
Upper respiratory tract infection		Pooled	11/48 [22.9]	4/45 [8.9]	2.6(0.9 to 7.5)	22.93	0.14(-0.01 to 0.29)	27.66
Upper respiratory	200mg	Winner, 2005[8]	22/112	8/50	1.2(0.6 to 2.6)	48.28	0.04(-0.09 to 0.16)	36.99

Appendix Table D52. Adverse effects with topiramate vs. placebo in children (pooled with random effects results from randomized controlled clinical trials) (continued)

Outcome	Dose	Reference, Risk of bias	Events/ Randomized [rate, %] with drug	Events/ Randomized [rate, %] with placebo	Relative risk (95% CI)	Weight	Absolute risk difference (95% CI)	Weight
tract infection		Medium	[19.6]	[16.0]				
Upper respiratory tract infection	200mg	Winner, 2006[15] Low	3/14 [21.4]	1/12 [8.3]	2.6(0.3 to 21.6)	5.8	0.13(-0.14 to 0.40)	8.24
Upper respiratory tract infection		Pooled	25/126 [19.8]	9/62 [14.5]	1.3(0.7 to 2.7)	54.08	0.05(-0.06 to 0.17)	45.23
Upper respiratory tract infection		**Pooled**	**48/221 [21.7]**	**17/152 [11.2]**	**1.8(1.1 to 3.1)**	**100**	**0.11(0.03 to 0.18)**	**100**
Weight decrease	50mg	Lewis, 2009[7] Low	10/35 [28.6]	7/33 [21.2]	1.3(0.6 to 3.1)	32.69	0.07(-0.13 to 0.28)	9.37
Weight decrease	50mg	Winner, 2006[15] Low	2/12 [16.7]	1/12 [8.3]	2.0(0.2 to 19.2)	4.51	0.08(-0.18 to 0.35)	5.69
Weight decrease		Pooled	12/47 [25.5]	8/45 [17.8]	1.4(0.6 to 3.1)	37.2	0.08(-0.08 to 0.24)	15.06
Weight decrease	100mg	Lewis, 2009[7] Low	17/35 [48.6]	7/33 [21.2]	2.3(1.1 to 4.8)	42.12	0.27(0.06 to 0.49)	8.36
Weight decrease	100mg	Winner, 2006[15] Low	2/13 [15.4]	1/12 [8.3]	1.8(0.2 to 17.8)	4.49	0.07(-0.18 to 0.32)	6.23
Weight decrease		Pooled	19/48 [39.6]	8/45 [17.8]	2.2(1.1 to 4.5)	46.61	0.18(-0.02 to 0.38)	14.6
Weight decrease	200mg	Winner, 2005[8] Medium	11/112 [9.8]	2/50 [4.0]	2.5(0.6 to 10.7)	10.7	0.06(-0.02 to 0.14)	65.47
Weight decrease	200mg	Winner, 2006[15] Low	4/14 [28.6]	1/12 [8.3]	3.4(0.4 to 26.7)	5.49	0.20(-0.08 to 0.49)	4.87
Weight decrease		Pooled	15/126 [11.9]	3/62 [4.8]	2.8(0.8 to 9.1)	16.19	0.07(-0.01 to 0.14)	70.35
Weight decrease		**Pooled**	**46/221 [20.8]**	**19/152 [12.5]**	**2.0(1.2 to 3.2)**	**100**	**0.09(0.02 to 0.15)**	**100**

Outcome	Dose	Reference	Events/ Randomized [rate, %] with drug	Events/ Randomized [rate, %] with placebo	Peto Odds ratio (95% CI)	% Weight	Arcsine transformed risk difference (95% CI)	% Weight
Abdominal pain	50mg	Lewis, 2009[7] Low	3/35 [8.6]	3/33 [9.1]	0.9(0.2 to 5.0)	17.19	-0.01(-0.25 to 0.23)	19.47
Abdominal pain	50mg	Winner, 2006[15] Low	0/12 [0.0]	1/12 [8.3]	0.1(0.0 to 6.8)	3.1	-0.29(-0.69 to 0.11)	6.88
Abdominal pain		Pooled	3/47	4/45	0.7(0.2 to 3.2)	20.29	-0.10(-0.37 0.16)	26.34

Appendix Table D52. Adverse effects with topiramate vs. placebo in children (pooled with random effects results from randomized controlled clinical trials) (continued)

Outcome	Dose	Reference	Events/ Randomized [rate,%] with drug	Events/ Randomized [rate,%] with placebo	Peto Odds ratio (95% CI)	% Weight	Arcsine transformed risk difference (95% CI)	% Weight
Abdominal pain	100mg	Lewis, 2009[7] Low	[6.4] 5/35 [14.3]	[8.9] 3/33 [9.1]	1.6(0.4 to 7.1)	22.19	0.08(-0.16 to 0.32)	19.47
Abdominal pain	100mg	Winner, 2006[15] Low	2/13 [15.4]	1/12 [8.3]	1.9(0.2 to 20.2)	8.51	0.11(-0.28 to 0.50)	7.15
Abdominal pain		Pooled	7/48 [14.6]	4/45 [8.9]	1.7(0.5 to 5.9)	30.7	0.09(-0.11 to 0.29)	26.61
Abdominal pain	200mg	Winner, 2005[8] Medium	11/112 [9.8]	6/50 [12.0]	0.8(0.3 to 2.3)	40.5	-0.04(-0.20 to 0.13)	39.64
Abdominal pain	200mg	Winner, 2006[15] Low	2/14 [14.3]	1/12 [8.3]	1.8(0.2 to 18.7)	8.5	0.10(-0.29 to 0.48)	7.4
Abdominal pain		Pooled	13/126 [10.3]	7/62 [11.3]	0.9(0.3 to 2.4)	49.01	-0.02(-0.17 to 0.14)	47.05
Abdominal pain		Pooled	23/221 [10.4]	15/152 [9.9]	1.0(0.5 to 2.1)	100	-0.01(-0.11 to 0.10)	100
Anorexia	50mg	Lewis, 2009[7] Low	3/35 [8.6]	1/33 [3.0]	2.7(0.4 to 19.9)	12.95	0.12(-0.12 to 0.36)	19.47
Anorexia	50mg	Winner, 2006[15] Low	1/12 [8.3]	1/12 [8.3]	1.0(0.1 to 17.0)	6.49	0.00(-0.40 to 0.40)	6.88
Anorexia		Pooled	4/47 [8.5]	2/45 [4.4]	1.9(0.4 to 9.9)	19.43	0.09(-0.11 to 0.30)	26.34
Anorexia	100mg	Lewis, 2009[7] Low	4/35 [11.4]	1/33 [3.0]	3.4(0.6 to 20.6)	15.93	0.17(-0.07 to 0.41)	19.47
Anorexia	100mg	Winner, 2006[15] Low	1/13 [7.7]	1/12 [8.3]	0.9(0.1 to 15.6)	6.49	-0.01(-0.40 to 0.38)	7.15
Anorexia		Pooled	5/48 [10.4]	2/45 [4.4]	2.3(0.5 to 10.6)	22.42	0.12(-0.08 to 0.32)	26.61
Anorexia	200mg	Winner, 2005[8] Medium	15/112 [13.4]	4/50 [8.0]	1.7(0.6 to 4.7)	48.84	0.09(-0.08 to 0.25)	39.64
Anorexia	200mg	Winner, 2006[15] Low	2/14 [14.3]	1/12 [8.3]	1.8(0.2 to 18.7)	9.3	0.10(-0.29 to 0.48)	7.4
Anorexia		Pooled	17/126 [13.5]	5/62 [8.1]	1.7(0.7 to 4.4)	58.15	0.09(-0.06 to 0.24)	47.05
Anorexia		Pooled	26/221 [11.8]	9/152 [5.9]	1.9(0.9 to 3.8)	100	0.10(-0.01 to 0.20)	100
Dizziness	50mg	Lewis, 2009[7] Low	2/35 [5.7]	0/33 [0.0]	7.2(0.4 to 117.5)	18.55	0.24(0.00 to 0.48)	22.1
Dizziness	50mg	Winner, 2006[15]	0/12	2/12	0.1(0.0 to 2.1)	18.03	-0.42(-0.82 to -0.02)	18.43

Appendix Table D52. Adverse effects with topiramate vs. placebo in children (pooled with random effects results from randomized controlled clinical trials) (continued)

Outcome	Dose	Reference	Events/ Randomized [rate,%] with drug	Events/ Randomized [rate,%] with placebo	Peto Odds ratio (95% CI)	% Weight	Arcsine transformed risk difference (95% CI)	% Weight
Dizziness		Low	[0.0]	[16.7]				
Dizziness		Pooled	2/47 [4.3]	2/45 [4.4]	1.0(0.1 to 7.1)	36.58	-0.07(-0.72 to 0.58)	40.52
Dizziness	100mg	Lewis, 2009[7] Low	3/35 [8.6]	0/353 [0.0]	7.4(0.7 to 73.8)	27.4	0.30(0.06 to 0.54)	22.1
Dizziness	100mg	Winner, 2006[15] Low	0/13 [0.0]	2/12 [16.7]	0.1(0.0 to 1.9)	18.03	-0.42(-0.81 to -0.03)	18.61
Dizziness		Pooled	3/48 [6.3]	2/365 [4.4]	1.4(0.2 to 8.4)	45.44	-0.04(-0.75 to 0.66)	40.71
Dizziness	200mg	Winner, 2006[15] Low	0/14 [0.0]	2/12 [16.7]	0.1(0.0 to 1.8)	17.99	-0.42(-0.81 to -0.04)	18.77
Dizziness		Pooled	5/109 [4.6]	6/422 [5.9]	0.8(0.2 to 2.6)	100	-0.12(-0.46 to 0.22)	100
Fatigue	50mg	Lewis, 2009[7] Low	2/35 [5.7]	2/33 [6.1]	0.9(0.1 to 7.0)	15.62	-0.01(-0.25 to 0.23)	19.47
Fatigue	50mg	Winner, 2006[15] Low	0/12 [0.0]	1/12 [8.3]	0.1(0.0 to 6.8)	4.09	-0.29(-0.69 to 0.11)	6.88
Fatigue		Pooled	2/47 [4.3]	3/45 [6.7]	0.6(0.1 to 3.8)	19.71	-0.10(-0.37 to 0.16)	26.34
Fatigue	100mg	Lewis, 2009[7] Low	3/35 [8.6]	2/33 [6.1]	1.4(0.2 to 8.8)	19.22	0.05(-0.19 to 0.29)	19.47
Fatigue	100mg	Winner, 2006[15] Low	1/13 [7.7]	1/12 [8.3]	0.9(0.1 to 15.6)	7.83	-0.01(-0.40 to 0.38)	7.15
Fatigue		Pooled	4/48 [8.3]	3/45 [6.7]	1.3(0.3 to 5.8)	27.05	0.03(-0.17 to 0.24)	26.61
Fatigue	200mg	Winner, 2005[8] Medium	7/112 [6.3]	6/50 [12.0]	0.5(0.1 to 1.6)	42.01	-0.10(-0.27 to 0.07)	39.64
Fatigue	200mg	Winner, 2006[15] Low	2/14 [14.3]	1/12 [8.3]	1.8(0.2 to 18.7)	11.23	0.10(-0.29 to 0.48)	7.4
Fatigue		Pooled	9/126 [7.1]	7/62 [11.3]	0.6(0.2 to 1.8)	53.24	-0.07(-0.22 to 0.08)	47.05
Fatigue		Pooled	15/221 [6.8]	13/152 [8.6]	0.7(0.3 to 1.7)	100	-0.05(-0.15 to 0.06)	100
Injury	50mg	Lewis, 2009[7] Low	3/35 [8.6]	2/33 [6.1]	1.4(0.2 to 8.8)	17.42	0.05(-0.19 to 0.29)	19.47
Injury	50mg	Winner, 2006[15] Low	1/12 [8.3]	1/12 [8.3]	1.0(0.1 to 17.0)	7.09	0.00(-0.40 to 0.40)	6.88
Injury		Pooled	4/47	3/45	1.3(0.3 to 5.9)	24.52	0.04(-0.17 to 0.24)	26.34

Appendix Table D52. Adverse effects with topiramate vs. placebo in children (pooled with random effects results from randomized controlled clinical trials) (continued)

Outcome	Dose	Reference	Events/ Randomized [rate,%] with drug	Events/ Randomized [rate,%] with placebo	Peto Odds ratio (95% CI)	% Weight	Arcsine transformed risk difference (95% CI)	% Weight
			[8.5]	[6.7]				
Injury	100mg	Lewis, 2009[7] Low	4/35 [11.4]	2/33 [6.1]	1.9(0.4 to 10.2)	20.57	0.10(-0.14 to 0.33)	19.47
Injury	100mg	Winner, 2006[15] Low	1/13 [7.7]	1/12 [8.3]	0.9(0.1 to 15.6)	7.1	-0.01(-0.40 to 0.38)	7.15
Injury		Pooled	5/48 [10.4]	3/45 [6.7]	1.6(0.4 to 6.7)	27.67	0.07(-0.14 to 0.27)	26.61
Injury	200mg	Winner, 2005[8] Medium	8/112 [7.1]	6/50 [12.0]	0.5(0.2 to 1.8)	40.74	-0.08(-0.25 to 0.08)	39.64
Injury	200mg	Winner, 2006[15] Low	1/14 [7.1]	1/12 [8.3]	0.9(0.1 to 14.5)	7.08	-0.02(-0.41 to 0.36)	7.4
Injury		Pooled	9/126 [7.1]	7/62 [11.3]	0.6(0.2 to 1.7)	47.82	-0.07(-0.23 to 0.08)	47.05
Injury		Pooled	18/221 [8.1]	13/152 [8.6]	0.9(0.4 to 2.0)	100	-0.01(-0.11 to 0.10)	100
Mood problems	50mg	Winner, 2006[15] Low	0/12 [0.0]	2/12 [16.7]	0.1(0.0 to 2.1)	22.33	-0.42(-0.82 to -0.02)	17.27
Mood problems	50mg	20159428 Low	1/35 [2.9]	0/33 [0.0]	7.0(0.1 to 352.3)	11.66	0.17(-0.07 to 0.41)	23.68
Mood problems		Pooled	1/47 [2.1]	2/45 [4.4]	0.5(0.1 to 4.9)	33.99	-0.10(-0.68 to 0.47)	40.96
Mood problems	100mg	Winner, 2006[15] Low	0/13 [0.0]	2/12 [16.7]	0.1(0.0 to 1.9)	22.33	-0.42(-0.81 to -0.03)	17.55
Mood problems	100mg	20159428 Low	1/35 [2.9]	0/33 [0.0]	7.0(0.1 to 352.3)	11.66	0.17(-0.07 to 0.41)	23.68
Mood problems		Pooled	1/48 [2.1]	2/45 [4.4]	0.5(0.0 to 4.6)	33.99	-0.10(-0.68 to 0.47)	41.24
Mood problems	200mg	Winner, 2006[15] Low	1/14 [7.1]	2/12 [16.7]	0.4(0.0 to 4.3)	32.02	-0.15(-0.54 to 0.24)	17.8
Mood problems		Pooled	3/109 [2.8]	6/102 [5.9]	0.5(0.1 to 1.7)	100	-0.09(-0.35 to 0.16)	100
Nausea	50mg	Lewis, 2009[7] Low	2/35 [5.7]	2/33 [6.1]	0.9(0.1 to 7.0)	24.14	-0.01(-0.25 to 0.23)	24.77
Nausea	100mg	Lewis, 2009[7] Low	3/35 [8.6]	2/33 [6.1]	1.4(0.2 to 8.8)	29.7	0.05(-0.19 to 0.29)	24.77
Nausea	200mg	Winner, 2005[8] Medium	6/112 [5.4]	3/50 [6.0]	0.9(0.2 to 3.8)	46.16	-0.01(-0.18 to 0.15)	50.45
Nausea		Pooled	11/182	7/116	1.0(0.4 to 2.8)	100	0.00(-0.12 to 0.12)	100

Appendix Table D52. Adverse effects with topiramate vs. placebo in children (pooled with random effects results from randomized controlled clinical trials) (continued)

Outcome	Dose	Reference	Events/Randomized [rate,%] with drug	Events/Randomized [rate,%] with placebo	Peto Odds ratio (95% CI)	% Weight	Arcsine transformed risk difference (95% CI)	% Weight
			[6.0]	[6.0]				
Paresthesia	50mg	Lewis, 2009[7] Low	8/35 [22.9]	1/33 [3.0]	5.5(1.4 to 22.1)	23.86	0.32(0.09 to 0.56)	19.47
Paresthesia	50mg	Winner, 2006[15] Low	1/12 [8.3]	2/12 [16.7]	0.5(0.0 to 5.1)	8.25	-0.13(-0.53 to 0.27)	6.88
Paresthesia		Pooled	9/47 [19.1]	3/45 [6.7]	2.9(0.9 to 9.7)	32.12	0.13(-0.31 to 0.57)	26.34
Paresthesia	100mg	Lewis, 2009[7] Low	4/35 [11.4]	1/33 [3.0]	3.4(0.6 to 20.6)	14.16	0.17(-0.07 to 0.41)	19.47
Paresthesia	100mg	Winner, 2006[15] Low	5/13 [38.5]	2/12 [16.7]	2.8(0.5 to 15.6)	15.79	0.25(-0.14 to 0.64)	7.15
Paresthesia		Pooled	9/48 [18.8]	3/45 [6.7]	3.1(0.9 to 10.6)	29.95	0.19(-0.01 to 0.39)	26.61
Paresthesia	200mg	Winner, 2005[8] Medium	9/112 [8.0]	0/50 [0.0]	4.6(1.1 to 19.5)	22	0.29(0.12 to 0.45)	39.64
Paresthesia	200mg	Winner, 2006[15] Low	5/14 [35.7]	2/12 [16.7]	2.5(0.5 to 14.0)	15.94	0.22(-0.17 to 0.61)	7.4
Paresthesia		**Pooled**	**14/126 [11.1]**	**2/62 [3.2]**	**3.6(1.2 to 10.8)**	**37.93**	**0.28(0.12 to 0.43)**	**47.05**
Paresthesia		**Pooled**	**32/221 [14.5]**	**8/152 [5.3]**	**3.2(1.6 to 6.3)**	**100**	**0.24(0.13 to 0.34)**	**100**
Sinusitis	50mg	Lewis, 2009[7] Low	2/35 [5.7]	1/33 [3.0]	1.9(0.2 to 18.6)	13.31	0.07(-0.17 to 0.30)	20.37
Sinusitis	50mg	Winner, 2006[15] Low	1/12 [8.3]	0/12 [0.0]	7.4(0.1 to 372.4)	4.58	0.29(-0.11 to 0.69)	9.07
Sinusitis		Pooled	3/47 [6.4]	1/45 [2.2]	2.7(0.4 to 19.3)	17.88	0.13(-0.08 to 0.33)	29.44
Sinusitis	100mg	Lewis, 2009[7] Low	1/35 [2.9]	1/33 [3.0]	0.9(0.1 to 15.4)	9.01	-0.01(-0.24 to 0.23)	20.37
Sinusitis	100mg	Winner, 2006[15] Low	1/13 [7.7]	0/12 [0.0]	6.8(0.1 to 345.9)	4.57	0.28(-0.11 to 0.67)	9.38
Sinusitis		Pooled	2/48 [4.2]	1/45 [2.2]	1.8(0.2 to 17.9)	13.58	0.09(-0.17 to 0.36)	29.75
Sinusitis	200mg	Winner, 2005[8] Medium	11/112 [9.8]	6/50 [12.0]	0.8(0.3 to 2.3)	59.8	-0.04(-0.20 to 0.13)	31.15
Sinusitis	200mg	Winner, 2006[15] Low	2/14 [14.3]	0/12 [0.0]	6.9(0.4 to 118.1)	8.73	0.39(0.00 to 0.77)	9.66
Sinusitis		Pooled	13/126	6/62	1.0(0.4 to 2.9)	68.54	0.14(-0.27 to 0.55)	40.81

Appendix Table D52. Adverse effects with topiramate vs. placebo in children (pooled with random effects results from randomized controlled clinical trials) (continued)

Outcome	Dose	Reference	Events/ Randomized [rate,%] with drug	Events/ Randomized [rate,%] with placebo	Peto Odds ratio (95% CI)	% Weight	Arcsine transformed risk difference (95% CI)	% Weight
Sinusitis		Pooled	18/221 [10.3] [8.1]	8/152 [9.7] [5.3]	1.3(0.6 to 3.1)	100	0.09(-0.04 to 0.22)	100
Somnolence	50mg	Winner, 2006[15] Low	1/12 [8.3]	1/12 [8.3]	1.0(0.1 to 17.0)	10.58	0.00(-0.40 to 0.40)	8.54
Somnolence	100mg	Lewis, 2009[7] Low	2/35 [5.7]	0/33 [0.0]	7.2(0.4 to 117.5)	10.89	0.24(0.00 to 0.48)	24.17
Somnolence	100mg	Winner, 2006[15] Low	1/13 [7.7]	1/12 [8.3]	0.9(0.1 to 15.6)	10.58	-0.01(-0.40 to 0.38)	8.87
Somnolence		Pooled	3/48 [6.3]	1/45 [2.2]	2.6(0.4 to 19.1)	21.47	0.17(-0.06 to 0.39)	33.05
Somnolence	200mg	Winner, 2005[8] Medium	9/112 [8.0]	3/50 [6.0]	1.3(0.4 to 4.8)	52.78	0.04(-0.13 to 0.21)	49.23
Somnolence	200mg	Winner, 2006[15] Low	2/14 [14.3]	1/12 [8.3]	1.8(0.2 to 18.7)	15.17	0.10(-0.29 to 0.48)	9.19
Somnolence		Pooled	11/126 [8.7]	4/62 [6.5]	1.4(0.5 to 4.4)	67.95	0.05(-0.10 to 0.20)	58.42
Somnolence		Pooled	15/186 [8.1]	6/119 [5.0]	1.6(0.6 to 3.9)	100	0.09(-0.03 to 0.20)	100
Upper respiratory tract infection	50mg	Lewis, 2009[7] Low	7/35 [20.0]	3/33 [9.1]	2.4(0.6 to 8.9)	17.07	0.16(-0.08 to 0.40)	19.47
Upper respiratory tract infection	50mg	Winner, 2006[15] Low	5/12 [41.7]	1/12 [8.3]	5.5(0.9 to 33.5)	9.26	0.41(0.01 to 0.81)	6.88
Upper respiratory tract infection		**Pooled**	**12/47 [25.5]**	**4/45 [8.9]**	**3.2(1.1 to 9.3)**	**26.33**	**0.23(0.01 to 0.45)**	**26.34**
Upper respiratory tract infection	100mg	Lewis, 2009[7] Low	8/35 [22.9]	3/33 [9.1]	2.7(0.8 to 9.8)	18.45	0.19(-0.05 to 0.43)	19.47
Upper respiratory tract infection	100mg	Winner, 2006[15] Low	3/13 [23.1]	1/12 [8.3]	2.9(0.4 to 23.3)	6.89	0.21(-0.18 to 0.60)	7.15
Upper respiratory tract infection		Pooled	11/48 [22.9]	4/45 [8.9]	2.8(0.9 to 8.2)	25.34	0.20(-0.01 to 0.40)	26.61
Upper respiratory tract infection	200mg	Winner, 2005[8] Medium	22/112 [19.6]	8/50 [16.0]	1.3(0.5 to 3.0)	41.42	0.05(-0.12 to 0.21)	39.64
Upper respiratory tract infection	200mg	Winner, 2006[15] Low	3/14 [21.4]	1/12 [8.3]	2.6(0.3 to 21.4)	6.9	0.19(-0.20 to 0.57)	7.4
Upper respiratory tract infection		Pooled	25/126 [19.8]	9/62 [14.5]	1.4(0.6 to 3.1)	48.33	0.07(-0.08 to 0.22)	47.05

Appendix Table D52. Adverse effects with topiramate vs. placebo in children (pooled with random effects results from randomized controlled clinical trials) (continued)

Outcome	Dose	Reference	Events/Randomized [rate,%] with drug	Events/Randomized [rate,%] with placebo	Peto Odds ratio (95% CI)	% Weight	Arcsine transformed risk difference (95% CI)	% Weight
Upper respiratory tract infection		Pooled	**48/221 [21.7]**	**17/152 [11.2]**	**2.1(1.2 to 3.6)**	**100**	**0.14(0.04 to 0.25)**	**100**
Weight decrease	50mg	Lewis, 2009[7] Low	10/35 [28.6]	7/33 [21.2]	1.5(0.5 to 4.4)	26.6	0.09(-0.15 to 0.32)	19.47
Weight decrease	50mg	Winner, 2006[15] Low	2/12 [16.7]	1/12 [8.3]	2.1(0.2 to 22.2)	5.64	0.13(-0.27 to 0.53)	6.88
Weight decrease		Pooled	12/47 [25.5]	8/45 [17.8]	1.6(0.6 to 4.2)	32.24	0.10(-0.11 to 0.30)	26.34
Weight decrease	100mg	Lewis, 2009[7] Low	17/35 [48.6]	7/33 [21.2]	3.3(1.2 to 8.7)	32.4	0.29(0.06 to 0.53)	19.47
Weight decrease	100mg	Winner, 2006[15] Low	2/13 [15.4]	1/12 [8.3]	1.9(0.2 to 20.2)	5.65	0.11(-0.28 to 0.50)	7.15
Weight decrease		Pooled	**19/48 [39.6]**	**8/45 [17.8]**	**3.0(1.2 to 7.5)**	**38.05**	**0.24(0.04 to 0.45)**	**26.61**
Weight decrease	200mg	Winner, 2005[8] Medium	11/112 [9.8]	2/50 [4.0]	2.2(0.6 to 7.4)	21.13	0.12(-0.05 to 0.28)	39.64
Weight decrease	200mg	Winner, 2006[15] Low	4/14 [28.6]	1/12 [8.3]	3.5(0.5 to 23.8)	8.59	0.27(-0.11 to 0.66)	7.4
Weight decrease		Pooled	15/126 [11.9]	3/62 [4.8]	2.5(0.9 to 7.0)	29.72	0.14(-0.01 to 0.30)	47.05
Weight decrease		Pooled	**46/221 [20.8]**	**19/152 [12.5]**	**2.3(1.3 to 4.0)**	**100**	**0.16(0.05 to 0.26)**	**100**

Outcome	Topiramate dose	Degree of freedom	Effect Measure	P	I-squared	Effect Measure	P	I-squared
Abdominal pain	50	1	Relative risk	0.556	0.00%	Risk difference	0.529	0.00%
Abdominal pain	100	1	Relative risk	0.905	0.00%	Risk difference	0.901	0.00%
Abdominal pain	200	1	Relative risk	0.556	0.00%	Risk difference	0.545	0.00%
Abdominal pain	Overall	5	Relative risk	0.905	0.00%	Risk difference	0.875	0.00%
Anorexia	50	1	Relative risk	0.555	0.00%	Risk difference	0.66	0.00%
Anorexia	100	1	Relative risk	0.419	0.00%	Risk difference	0.469	0.00%

Appendix Table D52. Adverse effects with topiramate vs. placebo in children (pooled with random effects results from randomized controlled clinical trials) (continued)

Outcome	Topiramate dose	Degree of freedom	Effect Measure	P	I-squared	Effect Measure	P	I-squared
Anorexia	200	1	Relative risk	0.985	0.00%	Risk difference	0.966	0.00%
Anorexia	Overall	5	Relative risk	0.957	0.00%	Risk difference	0.978	0.00%
Dizziness	50	1	Relative risk	0.14	54.10%	Risk difference	0.086	66.00%
Dizziness	100	1	Relative risk	0.091	64.90%	Risk difference	0.055	72.90%
Dizziness	Overall	4	Relative risk	0.187	35.10%	Risk difference	0.052	57.30%
Fatigue	50	1	Relative risk	0.576	0.00%	Risk difference	0.499	0.00%
Fatigue	100	1	Relative risk	0.792	0.00%	Risk difference	0.802	0.00%
Fatigue	200	1	Relative risk	0.35	0.00%	Risk difference	0.38	0.00%
Fatigue	Overall	5	Relative risk	0.871	0.00%	Absolute risk difference	0.858	0.00%
Injury	50	1	Relative risk	0.83	0.00%	Risk difference	0.846	0.00%
Injury	100	1	Relative risk	0.653	0.00%	Risk difference	0.639	0.00%

Bold = significant at 95% confidence level when 95% CI of absolute risk difference do not include 0

Appendix Table D53. Dose response effect on adverse effects with topiramate in children (results from randomized controlled clinical trials)

Compared doses	Type of outcome	Reference	Events/randomized with smaller dose	Events/randomized with larger dose	Relative risk (95% CI)	Absolute risk difference (95% CI)	Arcsine transformed Risk difference (95% CI)
50mg vs. 100mg	Abdominal pain	Winner, 2006[15]	0/12	2/13	0.2 (0.0 to 4.4)	-0.14 (-0.36 to 0.07)	-0.39 (-0.77 to 0.00)
50mg vs. 200mg	Abdominal pain	Winner, 2006[15]	0/12	2/14	0.2 (0.0 to 4.1)	-0.14 (-0.36 to 0.07)	-0.39 (-0.77 to -0.01)
100mg vs. 200mg	Abdominal pain	Winner, 2006[15]	2/13	2/14	1.0 (0.1 to 6.7)	0.00 (-0.11 to 0.11)	0.00 (-0.23 to 0.23)
50mg vs. 100mg	Abdominal pain	Lewis, 2009[7]	3/35	5/35	0.6 (0.2 to 2.3)	-0.06 (-0.21 to 0.09)	-0.09 (-0.32 to 0.14)
50mg vs. 100mg	Abnormal vision	Lewis, 2009[7]	1/35	2/35	0.5 (0.0 to 5.3)	-0.03 (-0.12 to 0.07)	-0.07 (-0.31 to 0.16)
50mg vs. 100mg	Allergy	Lewis, 2009[7]	0/35	2/35	0.2 (0.0 to 4.0)	-0.06 (-0.15 to 0.03)	-0.24 (-0.48 to -0.01)
50mg vs. 100mg	Anorexia	Winner, 2006[15]	1/12	1/13	1.0 (0.1 to 15.4)	0.00 (-0.08 to 0.08)	0.00 (-0.23 to 0.23)
50mg vs. 200mg	Anorexia	Winner, 2006[15]	1/12	2/14	0.5 (0.1 to 5.3)	-0.07 (-0.30 to 0.17)	-0.11 (-0.48 to 0.27)
100mg vs. 200mg	Anorexia	Winner, 2006[15]	1/13	2/14	0.5 (0.0 to 5.3)	-0.03 (-0.12 to 0.07)	-0.07 (-0.31 to 0.16)
50mg vs. 100mg	Anorexia	Lewis, 2009[7] Pandina, 2010[17]	3/35	4/35	0.8 (0.2 to 3.1)	-0.03 (-0.17 to 0.11)	-0.05 (-0.28 to 0.19)
50mg vs. 100mg	Any adverse event	Winner, 2006[15]	8/12	11/13	0.8 (0.5 to 1.4)	-0.12 (-0.46 to 0.22)	-0.13 (-0.52 to 0.25)
50mg vs. 200mg	Any adverse event	Winner, 2006[15]	8/12	12/14	0.7 (0.3 to 1.4)	-0.11 (-0.32 to 0.10)	-0.13 (-0.36 to 0.11)
50mg vs. 100mg	Any adverse event	Lewis, 2009[7]	26/35	26/35	1.0 (0.8 to 1.3)	0.00 (-0.20 to 0.20)	0.00 (-0.23 to 0.23)
100mg vs. 200mg	Any adverse event	Winner, 2006[15]	11/13	12/14	0.9 (0.5 to 1.8)	-0.03 (-0.25 to 0.19)	-0.03 (-0.26 to 0.20)
50mg vs. 100mg	Asthma	Lewis, 2009[7]	0/35	2/35	0.2 (0.0 to 4.0)	-0.06 (-0.15 to 0.03)	-0.24 (-0.48 to -0.01)
50mg vs. 100mg	Back pain	Lewis, 2009[7]	0/35	2/35	0.2 (0.0 to 4.0)	-0.06 (-0.15 to 0.03)	-0.24 (-0.48 to -0.01)
50mg vs. 100mg	Bronchitis	Winner, 2006[15]	0/12	1/13	0.4 (0.0 to 8.1)	-0.07 (-0.25 to 0.11)	-0.27 (-0.65 to 0.11)

Appendix Table D53. Dose response effect on adverse effects with topiramate in children (results from randomized controlled clinical trials) (continued)

Compared doses	Type of outcome	Reference	Events/ randomized with smaller dose	Events/ randomized with larger dose	Relative risk (95% CI)	Absolute risk difference (95% CI)	Arcsine transformed Risk difference (95% CI)
100mg vs. 200mg	Bronchitis	Winner, 2006[15]	1/13	0/14	3.0 (0.1 to 71.2)	0.03 (-0.05 to 0.10)	0.17 (-0.06 to 0.40)
50mg vs. 100mg	Conjunctivitis	Lewis, 2009[7]	3/35	1/35	3.0 (0.3 to 27.5)	0.06 (-0.05 to 0.17)	0.13 (-0.11 to 0.36)
50mg vs. 100mg	Cough	Lewis, 2009[7]	3/35	1/35	3.0 (0.3 to 27.5)	0.06 (-0.05 to 0.17)	0.13 (-0.11 to 0.36)
50mg vs. 100mg	Depression	Pandina, 2010[17]	1/35	0/35	3.2 (0.1 to 72.5)	0.08 (-0.12 to 0.28)	0.29 (-0.10 to 0.69)
50mg vs. 100mg	Diarrhea	Winner, 2006[15]	0/12	1/13	0.4 (0.0 to 8.7)	-0.07 (-0.26 to 0.11)	-0.27 (-0.66 to 0.11)
50mg vs. 200mg	Diarrhea	Winner, 2006[15]	0/12	1/14	0.4 (0.0 to 8.1)	-0.07 (-0.25 to 0.11)	-0.27 (-0.65 to 0.11)
100mg vs. 200mg	Diarrhea	Winner, 2006[15]	1/13	1/14	1.2 (0.1 to 16.7)	0.01 (-0.19 to 0.22)	0.02 (-0.36 to 0.41)
50mg vs. 200mg	Difficulty concentration/attention	Winner, 2006[15]	0/12	2/14	0.2 (0.0 to 4.1)	-0.14 (-0.36 to 0.07)	-0.39 (-0.77 to -0.01)
100mg vs. 200mg	Difficulty concentration/attention	Winner, 2006[15]	0/13	2/14	0.2 (0.0 to 4.4)	-0.14 (-0.36 to 0.07)	-0.39 (-0.77 to 0.00)
50mg vs. 200mg	Difficulty memory numbers	Winner, 2006[15]	0/12	1/14	0.4 (0.0 to 8.1)	-0.07 (-0.25 to 0.11)	-0.27 (-0.65 to 0.11)
100mg vs. 200mg	Difficulty memory numbers	Winner, 2006[15]	0/13	1/14	0.3 (0.0 to 7.9)	-0.03 (-0.10 to 0.05)	-0.17 (-0.40 to 0.06)
50mg vs. 100mg	Difficulty with concentration or attention	Pandina, 2010[17]	0/35	1/35	0.3 (0.0 to 7.9)	-0.03 (-0.10 to 0.05)	-0.17 (-0.40 to 0.06)
50mg vs. 100mg	Dizziness	Lewis, 2009[7] Pandina, 2010[17]	2/35	3/35	0.7 (0.1 to 3.7)	-0.03 (-0.15 to 0.09)	-0.06 (-0.29 to 0.18)
50mg vs. 100mg	Emotional lability	Pandina, 2010[17]	1/35	0/35	3.0 (0.1 to 71.2)	0.03 (-0.05 to 0.10)	0.17 (-0.06 to 0.40)
50mg vs. 100mg	Eye pain	Lewis, 2009[7]	1/35	1/35	1.0 (0.1 to 15.4)	0.00 (-0.08 to 0.08)	0.00 (-0.23 to 0.23)
50mg vs. 100mg	Fatigue	Winner, 2006[15]	0/12	1/13	0.3 (0.0 to 7.9)	-0.03 (-0.10 to 0.05)	-0.17 (-0.40 to 0.06)
50mg s. 200mg	Fatigue	Winner, 2006[15]	0/12	2/14	0.2 (0.0 to 4.0)	-0.06 (-0.15 to 0.03)	-0.24 (-0.48 to -0.01)

Appendix Table D53. Dose response effect on adverse effects with topiramate in children (results from randomized controlled clinical trials) (continued)

Compared doses	Type of outcome	Reference	Events/randomized with smaller dose	Events/randomized with larger dose	Relative risk (95% CI)	Absolute risk difference (95% CI)	Arcsine transformed Risk difference (95% CI)
50mg vs. 100mg	Fatigue	Lewis, 2009[7] Pandina, 2010[17]	2/35	3/35	0.7 (0.1 to 3.7)	-0.03 (-0.15 to 0.09)	-0.06 (-0.29 to 0.18)
100mg vs. 200mg	Fatigue	Winner, 2006[15]	1/13	2/14	0.5 (0.0 to 5.3)	-0.03 (-0.12 to 0.07)	-0.07 (-0.31 to 0.16)
50mg vs. 100mg	Fever	Lewis, 2009[7]	2/35	2/35	1.0 (0.1 to 6.7)	0.00 (-0.11 to 0.11)	0.00 (-0.23 to 0.23)
50mg vs. 100mg	Infection, viral	Winner, 2006[15]	1/12	1/13	1.2 (0.1 to 16.7)	0.01 (-0.19 to 0.22)	0.02 (-0.36 to 0.41)
50mg vs. 200mg	Infection, viral	Winner, 2006[15]	1/12	2/14	0.5 (0.0 to 5.3)	-0.03 (-0.12 to 0.07)	-0.07 (-0.31 to 0.16)
50mg vs. 100mg	Infection, viral	Lewis, 2009[7]	1/35	3/35	0.3 (0.0 to 3.1)	-0.06 (-0.17 to 0.05)	-0.13 (-0.36 to 0.11)
100mg vs. 200mg	Infection, viral	Winner, 2006[15]	1/13	2/14	0.5 (0.1 to 5.2)	-0.07 (-0.32 to 0.18)	-0.11 (-0.50 to 0.28)
50mg vs. 100mg	Injury	Winner, 2006[15]	1/12	1/13	1.2 (0.1 to 16.7)	0.01 (-0.19 to 0.22)	0.02 (-0.36 to 0.41)
50mg vs. 200mg	Injury	Winner, 2006[15]	1/12	1/14	1.1 (0.1 to 15.5)	0.01 (-0.19 to 0.20)	0.01 (-0.37 to 0.39)
100mg vs. 200mg	Injury	Winner, 2006[15]	1/13	1/14	1.0 (0.1 to 15.4)	0.00 (-0.08 to 0.08)	0.00 (-0.23 to 0.23)
50mg vs. 100mg	Injury	Lewis, 2009[7]	3/35	4/35	0.8 (0.2 to 3.1)	-0.03 (-0.17 to 0.11)	-0.05 (-0.28 to 0.19)
50mg vs. 100mg	Insomnia	Lewis, 2009[7] Pandina, 2010[17]	3/35	1/35	3.0 (0.3 to 27.5)	0.06 (-0.05 to 0.17)	0.13 (-0.11 to 0.36)
50mg vs. 200mg	Language problems	Winner, 2006[15]	0/12	2/14	0.2 (0.0 to 4.1)	-0.14 (-0.36 to 0.07)	-0.39 (-0.77 to -0.01)
100mg vs. 200mg	Language problems	Winner, 2006[15]	0/13	2/14	0.2 (0.0 to 4.0)	-0.06 (-0.15 to 0.03)	-0.24 (-0.48 to -0.01)
50mg vs. 100mg	Mood problems	Pandina, 2010[17]	1/35	1/35	1.2 (0.1 to 16.7)	0.01 (-0.19 to 0.22)	0.02 (-0.36 to 0.41)
50mg vs. 200mg	Mood problems	Winner, 2006[15]	0/12	1/14	0.4 (0.0 to 8.1)	-0.07 (-0.25 to 0.11)	-0.27 (-0.65 to 0.11)
100mg vs. 200mg	Mood problems	Winner, 2006[15]	0/13	1/14	0.3 (0.0 to 7.9)	-0.03 (-0.10 to 0.05)	-0.17 (-0.40 to 0.06)
50mg vs. 100mg	Nausea	Lewis, 2009[7]	2/35	3/35	0.7 (0.1 to 3.7)	-0.03 (-0.15 to 0.09)	-0.06 (-0.29 to 0.18)

Appendix Table D53. Dose response effect on adverse effects with topiramate in children (results from randomized controlled clinical trials) (continued)

Compared doses	Type of outcome	Reference	Events/ randomized with smaller dose	Events/ randomized with larger dose	Relative risk (95% CI)	Absolute risk difference (95% CI)	Arcsine transformed Risk difference (95% CI)
50mg vs. 100mg	Nervousness	Lewis, 2009[7] Pandina, 2010[17]	2/35	1/35	2.0 (0.2 to 21.1)	0.03 (-0.07 to 0.12)	0.07 (-0.16 to 0.31)
50mg vs. 100mg	Paresthesia	Winner, 2006[15]	1/12	5/13	0.2 (0.0 to 1.7)	-0.27 (-0.57 to 0.02)	-0.35 (-0.73 to 0.04)
50mg vs. 200mg	Paresthesia	Winner, 2006[15]	1/12	5/14	0.2 (0.0 to 1.6)	-0.28 (-0.57 to 0.01)	-0.36 (-0.74 to 0.02)
100mg vs. 200mg	Paresthesia	Winner, 2006[15]	5/13	5/14	1.0 (0.3 to 3.2)	0.00 (-0.16 to 0.16)	0.00 (-0.23 to 0.23)
50mg vs. 100mg	Paresthesia	Lewis, 2009[7]	8/35	4/35	2.0 (0.7 to 6.0)	0.11 (-0.06 to 0.29)	0.15 (-0.08 to 0.39)
50mg vs. 100mg	Pharyngitis	Lewis, 2009[7]	1/35	3/35	0.3 (0.0 to 3.1)	-0.06 (-0.17 to 0.05)	-0.13 (-0.36 to 0.11)
50mg vs. 100mg	Pneumonia	Lewis, 2009[7]	0/35	2/35	0.2 (0.0 to 4.0)	-0.06 (-0.15 to 0.03)	-0.24 (-0.48 to -0.01)
50mg vs. 100mg	Psychomotor slowing	Winner, 2006[15]	1/12	0/13	3.5 (0.2 to 77.9)	0.08 (-0.11 to 0.28)	0.29 (-0.09 to 0.68)
50mg vs. 200mg	Psychomotor slowing	Winner, 2006[15]	1/12	1/14	1.1 (0.1 to 15.5)	0.01 (-0.19 to 0.20)	0.01 (-0.37 to 0.39)
100mg vs. 200mg	Psychomotor slowing	Winner, 2006[15]	0/13	1/14	0.3 (0.0 to 7.9)	-0.03 (-0.10 to 0.05)	-0.17 (-0.40 to 0.06)
50mg vs. 100mg	Rhinitis	Lewis, 2009[7]	3/35	2/35	1.5 (0.3 to 8.4)	0.03 (-0.09 to 0.15)	0.06 (-0.18 to 0.29)
50mg vs. 100mg	Sinusitis	Winner, 2006[15]	1/12	1/13	1.2 (0.1 to 16.7)	0.01 (-0.19 to 0.22)	0.02 (-0.36 to 0.41)
50mg vs. 200mg	Sinusitis	Winner, 2006[15]	1/12	2/14	0.5 (0.1 to 5.3)	-0.07 (-0.30 to 0.17)	-0.11 (-0.48 to 0.27)
100mg vs. 200mg	Sinusitis	Winner, 2006[15]	1/13	2/14	0.5 (0.0 to 5.3)	-0.03 (-0.12 to 0.07)	-0.07 (-0.31 to 0.16)
50mg vs. 100mg	Sinusitis	Lewis, 2009[7]	2/35	1/35	2.0 (0.2 to 21.1)	0.03 (-0.07 to 0.12)	0.07 (-0.16 to 0.31)
50mg vs. 100mg	Somnolence	Winner, 2006[15]	1/12	1/13	1.0 (0.1 to 15.4)	0.00 (-0.08 to 0.08)	0.00 (-0.23 to 0.23)
50mg vs. 200mg	Somnolence	Winner, 2006[15]	1/12	2/14	0.5 (0.0 to 5.3)	-0.03 (-0.12 to 0.07)	-0.07 (-0.31 to 0.16)
50mg vs. 100mg	Somnolence	Lewis, 2009[7] Pandina, 2010[17]	0/35	2/35	0.2 (0.0 to 4.0)	-0.06 (-0.15 to 0.03)	-0.24 (-0.48 to -0.01)

Appendix Table D53. Dose response effect on adverse effects with topiramate in children (results from randomized controlled clinical trials) (continued)

Compared doses	Type of outcome	Reference	Events/ randomized with smaller dose	Events/ randomized with larger dose	Relative risk (95% CI)	Absolute risk difference (95% CI)	Arcsine transformed Risk difference (95% CI)
100mg vs. 200mg	Somnolence	Winner, 2006[15]	1/13	2/14	0.5 (0.0 to 5.3)	-0.03 (-0.12 to 0.07)	-0.07 (-0.31 to 0.16)
50mg vs. 100mg	Taste perversion	Lewis, 2009[7]	1/35	3/35	0.3 (0.0 to 3.1)	-0.06 (-0.17 to 0.05)	-0.13 (-0.36 to 0.11)
50mg vs. 100mg	Upper respiratory tract infection	Winner, 2006[15]	5/12	3/13	1.9 (0.6 to 6.5)	0.20 (-0.15 to 0.55)	0.22 (-0.17 to 0.61)
50mg vs. 200mg	Upper respiratory tract infection	Winner, 2006[15]	5/12	3/14	1.8 (0.5 to 6.1)	0.17 (-0.17 to 0.51)	0.19 (-0.19 to 0.57)
100mg vs. 200mg	Upper respiratory tract infection	Winner, 2006[15]	3/13	3/14	1.0 (0.2 to 4.6)	0.00 (-0.13 to 0.13)	0.00 (-0.23 to 0.23)
50mg vs. 100mg	Upper respiratory tract infection	Lewis, 2009[7]	7/35	8/35	0.9 (0.4 to 2.2)	-0.03 (-0.22 to 0.16)	-0.03 (-0.27 to 0.20)
50mg vs. 100mg	Vomiting	Lewis, 2009[7]	0/35	2/35	0.2 (0.0 to 4.0)	-0.06 (-0.15 to 0.03)	-0.24 (-0.48 to -0.01)
50mg vs. 100mg	Weight decrease	Winner, 2006[15]	2/12	2/13	1.2 (0.2 to 7.1)	0.02 (-0.26 to 0.30)	0.03 (-0.35 to 0.42)
50mg vs. 200mg	Weight decrease	Winner, 2006[15]	2/12	4/14	0.5 (0.1 to 2.6)	-0.06 (-0.19 to 0.07)	-0.10 (-0.34 to 0.13)
50mg vs. 100mg	Weight decrease	Lewis, 2009[7]	10/35	17/35	0.6 (0.3 to 1.1)	-0.20 (-0.42 to 0.02)	-0.21 (-0.44 to 0.03)
100mg vs. 200mg	Weight decrease	Winner, 2006[15]	2/13	4/14	0.5 (0.1 to 2.5)	-0.13 (-0.44 to 0.18)	-0.16 (-0.54 to 0.22)

Appendix Table D54. Strength of evidence that divalproex sodium resulted in treatment discontinuation due to lack of efficacy (results from randomized controlled clinical trial)[5]

Dose	Rate, %	RCTs	Children	Directness	Risk of bias	Consistency	Precision	Dose response	Strength of evidence	Conclusion
1000mg	0.0 [1.4]	1	148	Yes	Low	Not applicable	No	Not applicable	Low	Divalproex sodium 1000mg resulted in greater rates of treatment discontinuation due to lack of efficacy vs. placebo, the data is sparse
250mg	1.2 [1.4]	1	156	Yes	Low	Not applicable	No	Not applicable	Low	Divalproex sodium 250mg did not result in greater rates of treatment discontinuation due to lack of efficacy vs. placebo, the data is sparse
500mg	4.1 [1.4]	1	147	Yes	Low	Not applicable	No	Not applicable	Low	Divalproex sodium 500mg did not result in greater rates of treatment discontinuation due to lack of efficacy vs. placebo, the data is sparse

Appendix Table D55. Adverse effects with divalproex sodium vs. placebo in children (results from randomized controlled clinical trial reviewed by the FDA[6] and published as a journal article[5])

Outcome	Dose	Reference, Risk of bias	Events/randomized [rate, %] with drug	Events/randomized [rate, %] with placebo	Relative risk (95% CI)	Absolute risk difference (95% CI)
Any adverse event	1000mg	Apostol, 2008[5] Low	48/75 [64.0]	42/73 [57.5]	1.1 (0.9 to 1.4)	0.07 (-0.09 to 0.22)
	250mg	Apostol, 2008[5] Low	53/83 [63.9]	42/73 [57.5]	1.1 (0.9 to 1.4)	0.06 (-0.09 to 0.22)
	500mg	Apostol, 2008[5] Low	53/74 [71.6]	42/73 [57.5]	1.2 (1.0 to 1.6)	0.14 (-0.01 to 0.29)
Treatment discontinuation due to adverse events	**1000mg**	**Apostol, 2008[5] Low**	**7/75 [9.3]**	**1/73 [1.4]**	**6.8 (0.9 to 54.0)**	**0.08 (0.01 to 0.15)**
	250mg	Apostol, 2008[5] Low	2/83 [2.4]	1/73 [1.4]	1.8 (0.2 to 19.0)	0.01 (-0.03 to 0.05)
	500mg	Apostol, 2008[5] Low	0/74 [0.0]	1/73 [1.4]	0.3 (0.0 to 7.9)	-0.01 (-0.05 to 0.02)

Bold = significant at 95% confidence level 1 when 95% CI of absolute risk difference do not include 0

Appendix Table D56. Adverse effects with divalproex sodium vs. placebo in children (results from low risk of bias randomized controlled clinical trial)[5]

Outcome	Dose	Events/ randomized [rate, %] with drug	Events/ randomized [rate, %] with placebo	Relative risk (95% CI)	Absolute risk difference (95% CI)
Abdominal pain	1000mg	3/75 [4.0]	1/73 [1.4]	2.9 (0.3 to 27.4)	0.03 (-0.03 to 0.08)
Abdominal pain	250mg	1/83 [1.2]	1/73 [1.4]	0.9 (0.1 to 13.8)	0.00 (-0.04 to 0.03)
Abdominal pain	500mg	6/74 [8.1]	1/73 [1.4]	5.9 (0.7 to 48.0)	0.07 (0.00 to 0.14)
Ammonia increased	1000mg	4/75 [5.3]	0/73 [0.0]	8.8 (0.5 to 159.9)	0.05 (0.00 to 0.11)
Ammonia increased	1000mg	8/75 [10.7]	5/73 [6.8]	1.6 (0.5 to 4.5)	0.04 (-0.05 to 0.13)
Ammonia increased	250mg	2/83 [2.4]	0/73 [0.0]	4.4 (0.2 to 90.3)	0.02 (-0.02 to 0.06)
Ammonia increased	250mg	4/83 [4.8]	5/73 [6.8]	0.7 (0.2 to 2.5)	-0.02 (-0.09 to 0.05)
Ammonia increased	500mg	1/74 [1.4]	0/73 [0.0]	3.0 (0.1 to 71.5)	0.01 (-0.02 to 0.05)
Ammonia increased	500mg	2/74 [2.7]	5/73 [6.8]	0.4 (0.1 to 2.0)	-0.04 (-0.11 to 0.03)
Cough	1000mg	2/75 [2.7]	3/73 [4.1]	0.6 (0.1 to 3.8)	-0.01 (-0.07 to 0.04)
Cough	250mg	1/83 [1.2]	3/73 [4.1]	0.3 (0.0 to 2.8)	-0.03 (-0.08 to 0.02)
Cough	500mg	4/74 [5.4]	3/73 [4.1]	1.3 (0.3 to 5.7)	0.01 (-0.06 to 0.08)
Discontinued due to lack of efficacy	1000mg	0/75 [0.0]	1/73 [1.4]	0.3 (0.0 to 7.8)	-0.01 (-0.05 to 0.02)
Discontinued due to lack of efficacy	250mg	1/83 [1.2]	1/73 [1.4]	0.9 (0.1 to 13.8)	0.00 (-0.04 to 0.03)
Discontinued due to lack of efficacy	500mg	3/74 [4.1]	1/73 [1.4]	3.0 (0.3 to 27.8)	0.03 (-0.03 to 0.08)
Fatigue	1000mg	6/75 [8.0]	4/73 [5.5]	1.5 (0.4 to 5.0)	0.03 (-0.06 to 0.11)
Fatigue	250mg	1/83 [1.2]	4/73 [5.5]	0.2 (0.0 to 1.9)	-0.04 (-0.10 to 0.01)
Fatigue	500mg	1/74 [1.4]	4/73 [5.5]	0.2 (0.0 to 2.2)	-0.04 (-0.10 to 0.02)
Gastroenteritis viral	1000mg	4/75 [5.3]	1/73 [1.4]	3.9 (0.4 to 34.0)	0.04 (-0.02 to 0.10)
Gastroenteritis viral	250mg	4/83 [4.8]	1/73 [1.4]	3.5 (0.4 to 30.8)	0.03 (-0.02 to 0.09)
Gastroenteritis viral	500mg	1/74 [1.4]	1/73 [1.4]	1.0 (0.1 to 15.5)	0.00 (-0.04 to 0.04)
Influenza	1000mg	3/75 [4.0]	5/73 [6.8]	0.6 (0.1 to 2.4)	-0.03 (-0.10 to 0.04)
Influenza	250mg	1/83 [1.2]	5/73 [6.8]	0.2 (0.0 to 1.5)	-0.06 (-0.12 to 0.01)
Influenza	500mg	5/74 [6.8]	5/73 [6.8]	1.0 (0.3 to 3.3)	0.00 (-0.08 to 0.08)
Nasopharyngitis	1000mg	3/75 [4.0]	6/73 [8.2]	0.5 (0.1 to 1.9)	-0.04 (-0.12 to 0.03)
Nasopharyngitis	250mg	5/83 [6.0]	6/73 [8.2]	0.7 (0.2 to 2.3)	-0.02 (-0.10 to 0.06)
Nasopharyngitis	500mg	5/74 [6.8]	6/73 [8.2]	0.8 (0.3 to 2.6)	-0.01 (-0.10 to 0.07)
Nausea	1000mg	7/75 [9.3]	3/73 [4.1]	2.3 (0.6 to 8.4)	0.05 (-0.03 to 0.13)
Nausea	250mg	5/83 [6.0]	3/73 [4.1]	1.5 (0.4 to 5.9)	0.02 (-0.05 to 0.09)
Nausea	500mg	6/74 [8.1]	3/73 [4.1]	2.0 (0.5 to 7.6)	0.04 (-0.04 to 0.12)
Pharyngolaryngeal pain	1000mg	1/75 [1.3]	3/73 [4.1]	0.3 (0.0 to 3.0)	-0.03 (-0.08 to 0.02)
Pharyngolaryngeal pain	250mg	1/83 [1.2]	3/73 [4.1]	0.3 (0.0 to 2.8)	-0.03 (-0.08 to 0.02)
Pharyngolaryngeal pain	500mg	5/74 [6.8]	3/73 [4.1]	1.6 (0.4 to 6.6)	0.03 (-0.05 to 0.10)
Somnolence	1000mg	4/75 [5.3]	1/73 [1.4]	3.9 (0.4 to 34.0)	0.04 (-0.02 to 0.10)
Somnolence	250mg	2/83 [2.4]	1/73 [1.4]	1.8 (0.2 to 19.0)	0.01 (-0.03 to 0.05)
Somnolence	500mg	4/74 [5.4]	1/73 [1.4]	3.9 (0.5 to 34.5)	0.04 (-0.02 to 0.10)
Treatment discontinuation	1000mg	13/75 [17.3]	6/73 [8.2]	2.1 (0.8 to 5.3)	0.09 (-0.02 to 0.20)

D-91

Appendix Table D56. Adverse effects with divalproex sodium vs. placebo in children (results from low risk of bias randomized controlled clinical trial) (continued)

Outcome	Dose	Events/ randomized [rate, %] with drug	Events/ randomized [rate, %] with placebo	Relative risk (95% CI)	Absolute risk difference (95% CI)
Treatment discontinuation	250mg	8/83 [9.6]	6/73 [8.2]	1.2 (0.4 to 3.2)	0.01 (-0.08 to 0.10)
Treatment discontinuation	500mg	12/74 [16.2]	6/73 [8.2]	2.0 (0.8 to 5.0)	0.08 (-0.03 to 0.18)
Upper respiratory tract infection	1000mg	4/75 [5.3]	5/73 [6.8]	0.8 (0.2 to 2.8)	-0.02 (-0.09 to 0.06)
Upper respiratory tract infection	250mg	12/83 [14.5]	5/73 [6.8]	2.1 (0.8 to 5.7)	0.08 (-0.02 to 0.17)
Upper respiratory tract infection	500mg	3/74 [4.1]	5/73 [6.8]	0.6 (0.1 to 2.4)	-0.03 (-0.10 to 0.05)
Viral infection	1000mg	0/75 [0.0]	2/73 [2.7]	0.2 (0.0 to 4.0)	-0.03 (-0.07 to 0.02)
Viral infection	250mg	3/83 [3.6]	2/73 [2.7]	1.3 (0.2 to 7.7)	0.01 (-0.05 to 0.06)
Viral infection	500mg	4/74 [5.4]	2/73 [2.7]	2.0 (0.4 to 10.4)	0.03 (-0.04 to 0.09)
Vomiting	1000mg	3/75 [4.0]	1/73 [1.4]	2.9 (0.3 to 27.4)	0.03 (-0.03 to 0.08)
Vomiting	250mg	2/83 [2.4]	1/73 [1.4]	1.8 (0.2 to 19.0)	0.01 (-0.03 to 0.05)
Vomiting	500mg	4/74 [5.4]	1/73 [1.4]	3.9 (0.5 to 34.5)	0.04 (-0.02 to 0.10)
Weight gain	1000mg	5/75 [6.7]	1/73 [1.4]	4.9 (0.6 to 40.7)	0.05 (-0.01 to 0.12)
Weight gain	250mg	5/83 [6.0]	1/73 [1.4]	4.4 (0.5 to 36.8)	0.05 (-0.01 to 0.10)
Weight gain	500mg	1/74 [1.4]	1/73 [1.4]	1.0 (0.1 to 15.5)	0.00 (-0.04 to 0.04)

Appendix Table D57. Dose response in adverse effects with divalproex sodium in children (results from randomized controlled clinical trial)[5, 6]

Compared doses	Type of outcome	Reference	Events/ randomized with smaller dose	Events/ randomized with larger dose	Relative risk (95% CI)	Absolute risk difference (95% CI)	Arcsine transformed Risk difference (95% CI)
250mg vs. 500mg	Abdominal pain	Apostol, 2008[5]	1/83	6/74	0.1 (0.0 to 1.2)	-0.07 (-0.14 to 0.00)	-0.18 (-0.34 to -0.02)
250mg vs. 1000mg	Abdominal pain	Apostol, 2008[5]	1/83	3/75	0.3 (0.0 to 2.8)	-0.03 (-0.08 to 0.02)	-0.09 (-0.25 to 0.06)
500mg vs. 1000mg	Abdominal pain	Apostol, 2008[5]	6/74	3/75	2.0 (0.5 to 7.8)	0.04 (-0.04 to 0.12)	0.09 (-0.07 to 0.25)
250mg vs. 500mg	Ammonia increased	Apostol, 2008[5]	2/83	1/74	1.8 (0.2 to 19.3)	0.01 (-0.03 to 0.05)	0.04 (-0.12 to 0.20)
250mg vs. 500mg	Ammonia increased (>90 micromol/L)	Apostol, 2008[5]	4/83	2/74	1.8 (0.3 to 9.5)	0.02 (-0.04 to 0.08)	0.06 (-0.10 to 0.21)
250mg vs. 1000mg	Ammonia increased	Apostol, 2008[5]	2/83	4/75	0.5 (0.1 to 2.4)	-0.03 (-0.09 to 0.03)	-0.08 (-0.23 to 0.08)
250mg vs. 1000mg	Ammonia increased (>90 micromol/L)	Apostol, 2008[5]	4/83	8/75	0.5 (0.1 to 1.4)	-0.06 (-0.14 to 0.03)	-0.11 (-0.27 to 0.04)
500mg vs. 1000mg	Ammonia increased	Apostol, 2008[5]	1/74	4/75	0.3 (0.0 to 2.2)	-0.04 (-0.10 to 0.02)	-0.12 (-0.28 to 0.04)
500mg vs. 1000mg	Ammonia increased (>90 micromol/L)	Apostol, 2008[5]	2/74	8/75	0.3 (0.1 to 1.2)	-0.08 (-0.16 to 0.00)	-0.17 (-0.33 to -0.01)
250mg vs. 500mg	Any adverse event	Apostol, 2008[5]	53/83	53/74	0.9 (0.7 to 1.1)	-0.08 (-0.22 to 0.07)	-0.08 (-0.24 to 0.07)
250mg vs. 1000mg	Any adverse event	Apostol, 2008[5]	53/83	48/75	1.0 (0.8 to 1.3)	0.00 (-0.15 to 0.15)	0.00 (-0.16 to 0.15)
500mg vs. 1000mg	Any adverse event	Apostol, 2008[5]	53/74	48/75	1.1 (0.9 to 1.4)	0.08 (-0.07 to 0.23)	0.08 (-0.08 to 0.24)
250mg vs. 500mg	Cough	Apostol, 2008[5]	1/83	4/74	0.2 (0.0 to 1.9)	-0.04 (-0.10 to 0.01)	-0.12 (-0.28 to 0.03)
250mg vs. 1000mg	Cough	Apostol, 2008[5]	1/83	2/75	0.5 (0.0 to 4.9)	-0.01 (-0.06 to 0.03)	-0.05 (-0.21 to 0.10)
500mg vs. 1000mg	Cough	Apostol, 2008[5]	4/74	2/75	2.0 (0.4 to 10.7)	0.03 (-0.04 to 0.09)	0.07 (-0.09 to 0.23)
250mg vs. 500mg	Fatigue	Apostol, 2008[5]	1/83	1/74	0.9 (0.1 to 14.0)	0.00 (-0.04 to 0.03)	-0.01 (-0.16 to 0.15)
250mg vs. 1000mg	Fatigue	Apostol, 2008[5]	1/83	6/75	0.2 (0.0 to 1.2)	-0.07 (-0.13 to 0.00)	-0.18 (-0.33 to -0.02)
500mg vs. 1000mg	Fatigue	Apostol, 2008[5]	1/74	6/75	0.2 (0.0 to 1.4)	-0.07 (-0.13 to 0.00)	-0.17 (-0.33 to -0.01)

Appendix Table D57. Dose response in adverse effects with divalproex sodium in children (results from randomized controlled clinical trial) (continued)

Compared doses	Type of outcome	Reference	Events/randomized with smaller dose	Events/randomized with larger dose	Relative risk (95% CI)	Absolute risk difference (95% CI)	Arcsine transformed Risk difference (95% CI)
250mg vs. 500mg	Gastroenteritis viral	Apostol, 2008[5]	4/83	1/74	3.6 (0.4 to 31.2)	0.03 (-0.02 to 0.09)	0.10 (-0.05 to 0.26)
250mg vs. 1000mg	Gastroenteritis viral	Apostol, 2008[5]	4/83	4/75	0.9 (0.2 to 3.5)	-0.01 (-0.07 to 0.06)	-0.01 (-0.17 to 0.14)
500mg vs. 1000mg	Gastroenteritis viral	Apostol, 2008[5]	1/74	4/75	0.3 (0.0 to 2.2)	-0.04 (-0.10 to 0.02)	-0.12 (-0.28 to 0.04)
250mg vs. 500mg	Infection, viral	Apostol, 2008[5]	3/83	4/74	0.7 (0.2 to 2.9)	-0.02 (-0.08 to 0.05)	-0.04 (-0.20 to 0.11)
250mg vs. 1000mg	Infection, viral	Apostol, 2008[5]	3/83	0/75	6.3 (0.3 to 120.6)	0.04 (-0.01 to 0.08)	0.19 (0.04 to 0.35)
500mg vs. 1000mg	Infection, viral	Apostol, 2008[5]	4/74	0/75	9.1 (0.5 to 166.5)	0.05 (0.00 to 0.11)	0.23 (0.07 to 0.40)
250mg vs. 500mg	Influenza	Apostol, 2008[5]	1/83	5/74	0.2 (0.0 to 1.5)	-0.06 (-0.12 to 0.01)	-0.15 (-0.31 to 0.00)
250mg vs. 1000mg	Influenza	Apostol, 2008[5]	1/83	3/75	0.3 (0.0 to 2.8)	-0.03 (-0.08 to 0.02)	-0.09 (-0.25 to 0.06)
500mg vs. 1000mg	Influenza	Apostol, 2008[5]	5/74	3/75	1.7 (0.4 to 6.8)	0.03 (-0.04 to 0.10)	0.06 (-0.10 to 0.22)
250mg vs. 500mg	Nasopharyngitis	Apostol, 2008[5]	5/83	5/74	0.9 (0.3 to 3.0)	-0.01 (-0.08 to 0.07)	-0.01 (-0.17 to 0.14)
250mg vs. 1000mg	Nasopharyngitis	Apostol, 2008[5]	5/83	3/75	1.5 (0.4 to 6.1)	0.02 (-0.05 to 0.09)	0.05 (-0.11 to 0.20)
500mg vs. 1000mg	Nasopharyngitis	Apostol, 2008[5]	5/74	3/75	1.7 (0.4 to 6.8)	0.03 (-0.04 to 0.10)	0.06 (-0.10 to 0.22)
250mg vs. 500mg	Nausea	Apostol, 2008[5]	5/83	6/74	0.7 (0.2 to 2.3)	-0.02 (-0.10 to 0.06)	-0.04 (-0.20 to 0.12)
250mg vs. 1000mg	Nausea	Apostol, 2008[5]	5/83	7/75	0.6 (0.2 to 1.9)	-0.03 (-0.12 to 0.05)	-0.06 (-0.22 to 0.09)
500mg vs. 1000mg	Nausea	Apostol, 2008[5]	6/74	7/75	0.9 (0.3 to 2.5)	-0.01 (-0.10 to 0.08)	-0.02 (-0.18 to 0.14)
250mg vs. 500mg	Pharyngolaryngeal pain	Apostol, 2008[5]	1/83	5/74	0.2 (0.0 to 1.5)	-0.06 (-0.12 to 0.01)	-0.15 (-0.31 to 0.00)
250mg vs. 1000mg	Pharyngolaryngeal pain	Apostol, 2008[5]	1/83	1/75	0.9 (0.1 to 14.2)	0.00 (-0.04 to 0.03)	-0.01 (-0.16 to 0.15)
500mg vs. 1000mg	Pharyngolaryngeal pain	Apostol, 2008[5]	5/74	1/75	5.1 (0.6 to 42.3)	0.05 (-0.01 to 0.12)	0.15 (-0.01 to 0.31)
250mg vs. 500mg	Somnolence	Apostol, 2008[5]	2/83	4/74	0.4 (0.1 to 2.4)	-0.03 (-0.09 to 0.03)	-0.08 (-0.24 to 0.08)
250mg vs. 1000mg	Somnolence	Apostol, 2008[5]	2/83	4/75	0.5 (0.1 to 2.4)	-0.03 (-0.09 to 0.03)	-0.08 (-0.23 to 0.08)

Appendix Table D57. Dose response in adverse effects with divalproex sodium in children (results from randomized controlled clinical trial) (continued)

Compared doses	Type of outcome	Reference	Events/ randomized with smaller dose	Events/ randomized with larger dose	Relative risk (95% CI)	Absolute risk difference (95% CI)	Arcsine transformed Risk difference (95% CI)
500mg vs. 1000mg	Somnolence	Apostol, 2008[5]	4/74	4/75	1.0 (0.3 to 3.9)	0.00 (-0.07 to 0.07)	0.00 (-0.16 to 0.16)
250mg vs. 500mg	Upper respiratory tract infection	Apostol, 2008[5]	12/83	3/74	3.6 (1.0 to 12.1)	0.10 (0.02 to 0.19)	0.19 (0.03 to 0.34)
250mg vs. 1000mg	Upper respiratory tract infection	Apostol, 2008[5]	3/74	4/75	0.8 (0.2 to 3.3)	-0.01 (-0.08 to 0.06)	-0.03 (-0.19 to 0.13)
250mg vs. 1000mg	Upper respiratory tract infection	Apostol, 2008[5]	12/83	4/75	2.7 (0.9 to 8.0)	0.09 (0.00 to 0.18)	0.16 (0.00 to 0.31)
250mg vs. 500mg	Vomiting	Apostol, 2008[5]	2/83	4/74	0.4 (0.1 to 2.4)	-0.03 (-0.09 to 0.03)	-0.08 (-0.24 to 0.08)
250mg vs. 1000mg	Vomiting	Apostol, 2008[5]	2/83	3/75	0.6 (0.1 to 3.5)	-0.02 (-0.07 to 0.04)	-0.05 (-0.20 to 0.11)
500mg vs. 1000mg	Vomiting	Apostol, 2008[5]	4/74	3/75	1.4 (0.3 to 5.8)	0.01 (-0.05 to 0.08)	0.03 (-0.13 to 0.19)
250mg vs. 500mg	Weight increased	Apostol, 2008[5]	5/83	1/74	4.5 (0.5 to 37.3)	0.05 (-0.01 to 0.10)	0.13 (-0.03 to 0.29)
250mg vs. 1000mg	Weight increased	Apostol, 2008[5]	1/74	5/75	0.2 (0.0 to 1.7)	-0.05 (-0.12 to 0.01)	-0.14 (-0.31 to 0.02)
250mg vs. 1000mg	Weight increased	Apostol, 2008[5]	5/83	5/75	0.9 (0.3 to 3.0)	-0.01 (-0.08 to 0.07)	-0.01 (-0.17 to 0.14)
250mg vs. 500mg	Any adverse event	U.S. Food and Drug Administration[6]	54/83	53/74	0.9 (0.7 to 1.1)	-0.07 (-0.21 to 0.08)	0.00 (-0.23 to 0.08)
250mg vs. 1000mg	Any adverse event	U.S. Food and Drug Administration[6]	54/83	48/75	1.0 (0.8 to 1.3)	0.01 (-0.14 to 0.16)	0.00 (-0.15 to 0.17)
500mg vs. 1000mg	Any adverse event	U.S. Food and Drug Administration[6]	53/74	48/75	1.1 (0.9 to 1.4)	0.08 (-0.07 to 0.23)	0.00 (-0.07 to 0.25)
250mg vs. 1000mg	Serious adverse effects	U.S. Food and Drug Administration[6]	1/83	1/75	0.9 (0.1 to 14.2)	0.00 (-0.04 to 0.03)	-0.01 (-0.16 to 0.15)

Appendix Table D58. Adverse effects with propranolol, 80mg/day, vs. placebo in children (results from medium risk of bias randomized controlled clinical trial)[20]

Outcome	Events/ Randomized [rate, %] with drug	Events/ Randomized [rate, %] with placebo	Relative risk (95% CI)	Absolute risk difference (95% CI)
Abdominal pain	2/22 [9.1]	2/17 [11.8]	0.8 (0.1 to 4.9)	-0.03 (-0.22 to 0.17)
Amenorrhea	2/22 [9.1]	0/17 [0.0]	3.9 (0.2 to 76.5)	0.09 (-0.06 to 0.24)
Anorexia	1/22 [4.5]	0/17 [0.0]	2.3 (0.1 to 54.3)	0.05 (-0.08 to 0.17)
Depression	1/22 [4.5]	0/17 [0.0]	2.3 (0.1 to 54.3)	0.05 (-0.08 to 0.17)
Fatigue	3/22 [13.6]	0/17 [0.0]	5.5 (0.3 to 99.4)	0.14 (-0.03 to 0.30)
General worsening of behavior	2/22 [9.1]	0/17 [0.0]	3.9 (0.2 to 76.5)	0.09 (-0.06 to 0.24)
Increased appetite	3/22 [13.6]	1/17 [5.9]	2.3 (0.3 to 20.4)	0.08 (-0.10 to 0.26)
Menorrhagia	1/22 [4.5]	0/17 [0.0]	2.3 (0.1 to 54.3)	0.05 (-0.08 to 0.17)
Nausea	2/22 [9.1]	0/17 [0.0]	3.9 (0.2 to 76.5)	0.09 (-0.06 to 0.24)
Vomiting	1/22 [4.5]	0/17 [0.0]	2.3 (0.1 to 54.3)	0.05 (-0.08 to 0.17)
Weight gain	2/22 [9.1]	0/17 [0.0]	3.9 (0.2 to 76.5)	0.09 (-0.06 to 0.24)
Worsening of headache	2/22 [9.1]	1/17 [5.9]	1.5 (0.2 to 15.7)	0.03 (-0.13 to 0.20)

Appendix Table D59. Treatment discontinuation with antidepressant trazodone vs. placebo in children (results from low risk of bias randomized controlled clinical trial)[4]

Outcome	Dose	Events/Randomized [rate, %] with drug	Events/Randomized [rate, %] with placebo	Relative risk (95% CI)	Absolute risk difference (95% CI)
Treatment discontinuation	1mg/kg/day divided into 3 doses	2/20 [10.0]	3/20 [15.0]	0.7 (0.1 to 3.6)	-0.05 (-0.25 to 0.15)

Appendix Table D60. Adverse effects with clonidine, 25-50µg/day, vs. placebo in children (results from low risk of bias randomized controlled clinical trial)[2]

Outcome	Events/ Randomized [rate, %] with drug	Events/ Randomized [rate, %] with placebo	Relative risk (95% CI)	Absolute risk difference (95% CI)
Any adverse event	11/28 [39.3]	6/29 [20.7]	1.9 (0.8 to 4.4)	0.19 (-0.05 to 0.42)
Disturbed rhythms of the sleep-waking cycle and menstruation	1/28 [3.6]	0/29 [0.0]	3.1 (0.1 to 73.1)	0.04 (-0.06 to 0.13)
Fatigue	8/28 [28.6]	2/29 [6.9]	**4.1 (1.0 to 17.8)**	**0.22 (0.03 to 0.41)**
Irritability	0/28 [0.0]	1/29 [3.4]	0.3 (0.0 to 8.1)	-0.03 (-0.13 to 0.06)
Nausea	2/28 [7.1]	3/29 [10.3]	0.7 (0.1 to 3.8)	-0.03 (-0.18 to 0.11)
Pain in the right temporal region throughout treatment that ceased at the end of treatment	1/28 [3.6]	0/29 [0.0]	3.1 (0.1 to 73.1)	0.04 (-0.06 to 0.13)
Treatment discontinuation due to adverse events	1/28 [3.6]	0/29 [0.0]	3.1 (0.1 to 73.1)	0.04 (-0.06 to 0.13)

Bold = significant at 95% CI when 95% CI of absolute risk difference do not include 0

Appendix Table D61. Adverse effects with magnesium, 9mg/kg/day, vs. placebo in children (results from medium risk of bias randomized controlled clinical trials)[19]

Outcome	Events/ Randomized [rate, %] with drug	Events/ Randomized [rate, %] with placebo	Relative risk (95% CI)	Absolute risk difference (95% CI)
Diarrhea	11/58 [19.0]	4/60 [6.7]	2.8 (1.0 to 8.4)	0.12 (0.00 to 0.24)
Treatment discontinuation	16/58 [27.6]	16/60 [26.7]	1.0 (0.6 to 1.9)	0.01 (-0.15 to 0.17)
Treatment discontinuation because headache was resolved	1/58 [1.7]	2/60 [3.3]	0.5 (0.0 to 5.6)	-0.02 (-0.07 to 0.04)
Treatment discontinuation due to adverse events	3/58 [5.2]	1/60 [1.7]	3.1 (0.3 to 29.0)	0.04 (-0.03 to 0.10)

Appendix Table D62. Comparative safety of topiramate vs. sodium valproate in preventing migraine in children (results from a randomized controlled clinical trial with unclear risk of bias)[13]

Definition of the outcome	Active vs. control drug	Events/randomized in active control group Rate in active [control] group, %	Relative risk (95% CI)	Absolute risk difference (95% CI)
Nausea	Topiramate, 1-3mg/kg vs. Sodium valproate,10-15mg/kg	1/28 0/20 3.6 [0.0]	2.2 (0.1 to 50.7)	0.04 (-0.07 to 0.14)
Mood changes	Topiramate, 1-3mg/kg vs. Sodium valproate,10-15mg/kg	1/28 0/20 3.6 [0.0]	2.2 (0.1 to 50.7)	0.04 (-0.07 to 0.14)
Weight loss	Topiramate, 1-3mg/kg vs. Sodium valproate,10-15mg/kg	1/28 0/20 3.6 [0.0]	2.2 (0.1 to 50.7)	0.04 (-0.07 to 0.14)
Weakness	Topiramate, 1-3mg/kg vs. Sodium valproate,10-15mg/kg	1/28 0/20 3.6 [0.0]	2.2 (0.1 to 50.7)	0.04 (-0.07 to 0.14)
Raised liver transaminase	Topiramate, 1-3mg/kg vs. Sodium valproate,10-15mg/kg	1/28 0/20 3.6 [0.0]	2.2 (0.1 to 50.7)	0.04 (-0.07 to 0.14)
Drowsiness	Topiramate, 1-3mg/kg vs. Sodium valproate,10-15mg/kg	1/28 0/20 3.6 [0.0]	2.2 (0.1 to 50.7)	0.04 (-0.07 to 0.14)

References for Appendix D

1. Ludvigsson J. Propranolol used in prophylaxis of migraine in children. Acta neurologica Scandinavica; 1974. p. 109-15.

2. Sillanpää M. Clonidine prophylaxis of childhood migraine and other vascular headache. A double blind study of 57 children. Headache; 1977. p. 28-31.

3. Battistella PA, Ruffilli R, Moro R, et al. A placebo-controlled crossover trial of nimodipine in pediatric migraine. Headache. 1990 Apr;30(5):264-8. PMID 2191938.

4. Battistella PA, Ruffilli R, Cernetti R, et al. A placebo-controlled crossover trial using trazodone in pediatric migraine. Headache. 1993 Jan;33(1):36-9. PMID 8436497.

5. Apostol G, Cady RK, Laforet GA, et al. Divalproex extended-release in adolescent migraine prophylaxis: results of a randomized, double-blind, placebo-controlled study. Headache. 2008 Jul;48(7):1012-25. PMID 18705027.

6. U.S. Food and Drug Administration. Clinical Review of Divalproex Sodium. 2008.

7. Lewis D, Winner P, Saper J, et al. Randomized, double-blind, placebo-controlled study to evaluate the efficacy and safety of topiramate for migraine prevention in pediatric subjects 12 to 17 years of age. Pediatrics. 2009 Mar;123(3):924-34. PMID 19255022.

8. Winner P, Pearlman EM, Linder SL, et al. Topiramate for migraine prevention in children: a randomized, double-blind, placebo-controlled trial. Headache. 2005 Nov-Dec;45(10):1304-12. PMID 16324162.

9. Olness K, MacDonald JT, Uden DL. Comparison of self-hypnosis and propranolol in the treatment of juvenile classic migraine. Pediatrics. 1987 Apr;79(4):593-7. PMID 3822681.

10. Sorge F, Marano E. Flunarizine v. placebo in childhood migraine. A double-blind study. Cephalalgia. 1985 May;5 Suppl 2:145-8. PMID 2861907.

11. Ashrafi MR, Shabanian R, Zamani GR, et al. Sodium Valproate versus Propranolol in paediatric migraine prophylaxis. Eur J Paediatr Neurol. 2005;9(5):333-8. PMID 16120482.

12. Bidabadi E, Mashouf M. A randomized trial of propranolol versus sodium valproate for the prophylaxis of migraine in pediatric patients. Paediatric Drugs. 2010 Aug 1;12(4):269-75. PMID 20593910.

13. Unalp A, Uran N, Ozturk A. Comparison of the effectiveness of topiramate and sodium valproate in pediatric migraine. J Child Neurol. 2008 Dec;23(12):1377-81. PMID 19073842.

14. Sartory G, Muller B, Metsch J, et al. A comparison of psychological and pharmacological treatment of pediatric migraine. Behav Res Ther. 1998 Dec;36(12):1155-70. PMID 9745800.

15. Winner P, Gendolla A, Stayer C, et al. Topiramate for migraine prevention in adolescents: a pooled analysis of efficacy and safety. Headache. 2006 Nov-Dec;46(10):1503-10. PMID 17115983.

16. Lewis D, Paradiso E. A double-blind, dose comparison study of topiramate for prophylaxis of basilar-type migraine in children: a pilot study. Headache. 2007 Nov-Dec;47(10):1409-17. PMID 18052950.

17. Pandina GJ, Ness S, Polverejan E, et al. Cognitive effects of topiramate in migraine patients aged 12 through 17 years. Pediatr Neurol. 2010 Mar;42(3):187-95. PMID 20159428.

18. Trautmann E, Kroner-Herwig B. A randomized controlled trial of Internet-based self-help training for recurrent headache in childhood and adolescence. Behav Res Ther. 2010 Jan;48(1):28-37. PMID 19782343.

19. Wang F, Van Den Eeden SK, Ackerson LM, et al. Oral magnesium oxide prophylaxis of frequent migrainous headache in children: a randomized, double-blind, placebo-controlled trial. Headache. 2003 Jun;43(6):601-10. PMID 12786918.

20. Forsythe WI, Gillies D, Sills MA. Propanolol ('Inderal') in the treatment of childhood migraine. Developmental medicine and child neurology; 1984. p. 737-41.

21. Lewis DW, Diamond S, Scott D, et al. Prophylactic treatment of pediatric migraine. Headache. 2004 Mar;44(3):230-7. PMID 15012660.

22. Apostol G, Lewis DW, Laforet GA, et al. Divalproex sodium extended-release for the prophylaxis of migraine headache in adolescents: results of a stand-alone, long-term open-label safety study. Headache. 2009 Jan;49(1):45-53. PMID 19040679.

23. Pakalnis A, Greenberg G, Drake ME, Jr., et al. Pediatric migraine prophylaxis with divalproex. Journal of Child Neurology. 2001 Oct;16(10):731-4. PMID 11669346.

24. Pakalnis A, Kring D, Meier L. Levetiracetam prophylaxis in pediatric migraine--an open-label study. Headache. 2007 Mar;47(3):427-30. PMID 17371359.

25. Miller GS. Efficacy and safety of levetiracetam in pediatric migraine. Headache. 2004 Mar;44(3):238-43. PMID 15012661.

26. Cruz MJ, Valencia I, Legido A, et al. Efficacy and tolerability of topiramate in pediatric migraine. Pediatric Neurology. 2009 Sep;41(3):167-70. PMID 19664530.

27. Jurgens TP, Ihle K, Stork JH, et al. "Alice in Wonderland syndrome" associated with topiramate for migraine prevention. J Neurol Neurosurg Psychiatry. 2011 Feb;82(2):228-9. PMID 20571045.

28. Taylor LM, Farzam F, Cook AM, et al. Clinical utility of a continuous intravenous infusion of valproic acid in pediatric patients. Pharmacotherapy. 2007 Apr;27(4):519-25. PMID 17381378.

29. Chan VW, McCabe EJ, MacGregor DL. Botox treatment for migraine and chronic daily headache in adolescents. Journal of Neuroscience Nursing. 2009 Oct;41(5):235-43. PMID 19835236.

Appendix E. Excluded Studies

1. Why do placebos work in some kids with migraine. Child Health Alert 2008 Apr; 26:5; PMID: 18828187. *Comment*

2. Adam EI, Gore SM, Price WH. Double blind trial of clonidine in the treatment of migraine in a general practice. J R Coll Gen Pract 1978 Oct; 28(195):587-90; PMID: 368333. *Not eligible target population*

3. Adelman J, Freitag FG, Lainez M, et al. Analysis of safety and tolerability data obtained from over 1,500 patients receiving topiramate for migraine prevention in controlled trials. Pain Med 2008 Mar; 9(2):175-85; PMID: 18298700. *Not eligible target population*

4. Ahonen K, Hamalainen ML, Eerola M, et al. A randomized trial of rizatriptan in migraine attacks in children. Neurology 2006 Oct 10; 67(7):1135-40; PMID: 16943370. *Not eligible exposure*

5. Ahonen K, Hamalainen ML, Rantala H, et al. Nasal sumatriptan is effective in treatment of migraine attacks in children: A randomized trial. Neurology 2004 Mar 23; 62(6):883-7; PMID: 15037686. *Not eligible target population*

6. Albsoul-Younes AM, Salem HA, Ajlouni SF, et al. Topiramate slow dose titration: improved efficacy and tolerability. Pediatr Neurol 2004 Nov; 31(5):349-52; PMID: 15519117. *Not eligible target population*

7. Altinok D, Agarwal A, Ascadi G, et al. Pediatric hemiplegic migraine: susceptibility weighted and MR perfusion imaging abnormality. Pediatr Radiol 2010 Dec; 40(12):1958-61; PMID: 20821201. *Not eligible target population*

8. Anonymous. Prochlorperazine more effective than ketorolac for pediatric migraine. Journal of Family Practice; 2004: 444. *Not eligible target population*

9. Arnold LE, Amato A, Bozzolo H, et al. Acetyl-L-carnitine (ALC) in attention-deficit/hyperactivity disorder: a multi-site, placebo-controlled pilot trial. Journal of child and adolescent psychopharmacology; 2007: 791-802. *Not eligible target population*

10. Arruda MA, Guidetti V, Galli F, et al. Primary headaches in childhood--a population-based study. Cephalalgia 2010 Sep; 30(9):1056-64; PMID: 20713556. *Not eligible exposure*

11. Arthur GP, Hornabrook RW. The treatment of migraine with BC 105 (pizotifen): a double blind trial. The New Zealand medical journal; 1971: 5-9. *Not eligible exposure*

12. Aydin M, Kabakus N, Bozdag S, et al. Profile of children with migraine. Indian Journal of Pediatrics 2010 Nov; 77(11):1247-51; PMID: 20886317. *Not eligible target population*

13. Bademosi O, Osuntokun BO. Pizotifen in the management of migraine. Practitioner 1978 Feb; 220(1316):325-7; PMID: 345259. *Not eligible exposure*

14. Bakker MK, Kerstjens-Frederikse WS, Buys CH, et al. First-trimester use of paroxetine and congenital heart defects: a population-based case-control study. Birth Defects Res A Clin Mol Teratol 2010 Feb; 88(2):94-100; PMID: 19937603. *Not eligible exposure*

15. Barry J, von Baeyer CL. Brief cognitive-behavioral group treatment for children's headache. Clin J Pain 1997 Sep; 13(3):215-20; PMID: 9303253. *Not eligible exposure*

16. Baser O, Palmer L, Stephenson J. The estimation power of alternative comorbidity indices. Value in Health 2008 Sep-Oct; 11(5):946-55; PMID: 18489502. *Not eligible exposure*

17. Behan PO. Pizotifen in the treatment of severe recurrent headache single and divided dose therapy compared. The British journal of clinical practice; 1982: 13-7. *Not eligible exposure*

18. Besser RE, Stern CM. Raynaud phenomena and migraine in two children: inclusion within a family of related disorders. Acta Paediatrica 2005 Dec; 94(12):1860-2; PMID: 16421056. *Not eligible exposure*

19. Bigal ME, Borucho S, Serrano D, et al. The acute treatment of episodic and chronic migraine in the USA. Cephalalgia 2009 Aug; 29(8):891-7; PMID: 19222509. *Not eligible target population*

20. Bigal ME, Lipton RB, Winner P, et al. Migraine in adolescents: association with socioeconomic status and family history. Neurology 2007 Jul 3; 69(1):16-25; PMID: 17606878. *Not eligible outcomes*

21. Bigal ME, Rapoport AM, Sheftell FD, et al. Transformed migraine and medication overuse in a tertiary headache centre--clinical characteristics and treatment outcomes. Cephalalgia 2004 Jun; 24(6):483-90; PMID: 15154858. *Not eligible exposure*

22. Bigal ME, Sheftell FD, Tepper SJ, et al. Migraine days decline with duration of illness in adolescents with transformed migraine. Cephalalgia : an international journal of headache; 2005: 482-7. *Not eligible target population*

23. Bigal ME, Tsang A, Loder E, et al. Body mass index and episodic headaches: a population-based study. Archives of Internal Medicine 2007 Oct 8; 167(18):1964-70; PMID: 17923596. *Not eligible target population*

24. Bille B, Ludvigsson J, Sanner G. Prophylaxis of migraine in children. Headache; 1977: 61-3. *Not eligible exposure*

25. Boccia G, Del Giudice E, Crisanti AF, et al. Functional gastrointestinal disorders in migrainous children: efficacy of flunarizine. Cephalalgia 2006 Oct; 26(10):1214-9; PMID: 16961789. *Not eligible exposure*

26. Bottini F, Celle ME, Calevo MG, et al. Metabolic and genetic risk factors for migraine in children. Cephalalgia : an international journal of headache; 2006: 731-7. *Not eligible exposure*

27. Brandes JL, Saper JR, Diamond M, et al. Topiramate for migraine prevention: a randomized controlled trial. JAMA 2004 Feb 25; 291(8):965-73; PMID: 14982912. *Not eligible target population*

28. Briars GL, Travis SE, Anand B, et al. Weight gain with pizotifen therapy. Archives of Disease in Childhood 2008 Jul; 93(7):590-3; PMID: 18381348. *Not eligible exposure*

29. Brousseau D, Duffy S, Anderson A, et al. Migraines in the pediatric emergency department: A randomized, double blind trial of IV ketorolac versus IV prochlorperazine. Pediatric research; 2002: 101a. *Not eligible target population*

30. Brousseau DC, Duffy SJ, Anderson AC, et al. Treatment of pediatric migraine headaches: a randomized, double-blind trial of prochlorperazine versus ketorolac. Ann Emerg Med 2004 Feb; 43(2):256-62; PMID: 14747817. *Not eligible target population*

31. Bruni O, Galli F, Guidetti V. Sleep hygiene and migraine in children and adolescents. Cephalalgia 1999 Dec; 19 Suppl 25:57-9; PMID: 10668125. *Not eligible target population*

32. Burns C. Migraine in a rural practice (1958-1963). A five-year study of a controlled clinical trial. J Coll Gen Pract; 1965: 230-8. *Not eligible exposure*

33. Campos L, Diaz Gomez M, Ondiviela R, et al. Naproxen sodium in the treatment of otitis. Atencion Primaria; 1992: 314, 6-7. *Not eligible target population*

34. Caruso JM, Brown WD, Exil G, et al. The efficacy of divalproex sodium in the prophylactic treatment of children with migraine. Headache 2000 Sep; 40(8):672-6; PMID: 10971664. *Not eligible outcomes*

35. Castellana M, Carini C, Caprici G, et al. Calcium entry blockers in the treatment of primary headached in childhood: our experiecne with flunarizine and nimodipine. Paper presented at, 1989; Headache in children and adolescents. Proceedings of the First International Symposium on Headache in Children and Adolescents; 1988 May 19-20; Pavia Italy. *Not eligible exposure*

36. Chang CL, Donaghy M, Poulter N. Migraine and stroke in young women: case-control study. The World Health Organisation Collaborative Study of Cardiovascular Disease and Steroid Hormone Contraception. BMJ (Clinical research ed.); 1999: 13-8. *Not eligible target population*

37. Christensen MF. Double blind placebo controlled trial of pizotifen syrup in the treatment of abdominal migraine. Archives of disease in childhood; 1995: 183. *Not eligible exposure*

38. Christensen ML, Eades SK, Fuseau E, et al. Pharmacokinetics of naratriptan in adolescent subjects with a history of migraine. Journal of Clinical Pharmacology 2001 Feb; 41(2):170-5; PMID: 11210397. *Not eligible outcomes*

39. Christensen ML, Mottern RK, Jabbour JT, et al. Pharmacokinetics of sumatriptan nasal spray in children. Journal of Clinical Pharmacology 2004 Apr; 44(4):359-67; PMID: 15051742. *Not eligible outcomes*

40. Chun-Fai-Chan B, Koren G, Fayez I, et al. Pregnancy outcome of women exposed to bupropion during pregnancy: a prospective comparative study. Am J Obstet Gynecol 2005 Mar; 192(3):932-6; PMID: 15746694. *Not eligible exposure*

41. Cianchetti C, Serci MC, Pisano T, et al. Compression of superficial temporal arteries by a handmade device: a simple way to block or attenuate migraine attacks in children and adolescents. Journal of Child Neurology 2010 Jan; 25(1):67-70; PMID: 19525492. *Not eligible exposure*

42. Cohen D, Huinink S. Atypical antipsychotic-induced diabetes mellitus in child and adolescent psychiatry. CNS Drugs 2007; 21(12):1035-8; PMID: 18020482. *Comment*

43. Cologno D, Torelli P, Manzoni GC. Migraine with aura: a review of 81 patients at 10-20 years' follow-up. Cephalalgia : an international journal of headache; 1998: 690-6. *Not eligible exposure*

44. Conte Hr KTB. Psychotherapy for medically ill patients: review and critique of controlled studies. Review 35 refs. Psychosomatics; 1981: 285-90. *Not eligible target population*

45. Cunnington M, Ephross S, Churchill P. The safety of sumatriptan and naratriptan in pregnancy: what have we learned? Headache 2009 Nov-Dec; 49(10):1414-22; PMID: 19804390. *Not eligible exposure*

46. Cupini LM, Santorelli FM, Iani C, et al. Cyclic vomiting syndrome, migraine, and epilepsy: a common underlying disorder? Headache 2003 Apr; 43(4):407-9; PMID: 12656714. *Not eligible exposure*

47. Cuvellier J-C, Donnet A, Gu, et al. Treatment of primary headache in children: a multicenter hospital-based study in France. Journal of Headache & Pain 2009 Dec; 10(6):447-53; PMID: 19771388. *Not eligible exposure*

48. D'Andrea G, Cananzi AR, Grigoletto F, et al. The effect of dopamine receptor agonists on prolactin secretion in childhood migraine. Headache; 1988: 354-9. *Not eligible exposure*

49. Danesch U, Rittinghausen R. Safety of a patented special butterbur root extract for migraine prevention. Headache; 2003: 76-8. *Animal studies*

50. de Almeida R, x00E, o F, et al. Migraine with persistent visual aura: response to furosemide. Clinics (Sao Paulo, Brazil) 2009; 64(4):375-6; PMID: 19488599. *Not eligible exposure*

51. De Ciantis A, Muti M, Piccolini C, et al. A functional MRI study of language disturbances in subjects with migraine headache during treatment with topiramate. Neurological Sciences 2008 May; 29 Suppl 1:S141-3; PMID: 18545916. *Not eligible outcomes*

52. De Sanctis S, Grieco GS, Breda L, et al. Prolonged sporadic hemiplegic migraine associated with a novel de novo missense ATP1A2 gene mutation. Headache 2011 Mar; 51(3):447-50; PMID: 21352219. *Not eligible target population*

53. Del Bene E, Poggioni M, Michelacci S. Lisuride as a migraine prophylactic in children: an open clinical trial. Int J Clin Pharmacol Res 1983; 3(2):137-41; PMID: 6679514. *Not eligible exposure*

54. Di Rosa G, Attin, x00E, et al. Efficacy of folic acid in children with migraine, hyperhomocysteinemia and MTHFR polymorphisms. Headache 2007 Oct; 47(9):1342-4; PMID: 17927652. *Not eligible exposure*

55. Di Rosa G, Span, x00F, et al. Alternating hemiplegia of childhood successfully treated with topiramate: 18 months of follow-up. Neurology 2006 Jan 10; 66(1):146; PMID: 16401872. *Not eligible target population*

56. Diener H-C. Placebo effects in treating migraine and other headaches. Current Opinion in Investigational Drugs 2010 Jul; 11(7):735-9; PMID: 20597189. *Comment*

57. Dikel W, Olness K. Self-hypnosis, biofeedback, and voluntary peripheral temperature control in children. Pediatrics; 1980: 335-40. *Not eligible target population*

58. Ebinger F. Exteroceptive suppression of masseter muscle activity in juvenile migraineurs. Cephalalgia : an international journal of headache; 2006: 722-30. *Not eligible exposure*

59. Egger J, Carter C, Wilson J, et al. Food allergies and migraine in children. Monatsschrift fur Kinderheilkunde; 1983: 686. *Language*

60. Egger J, Carter CH, Soothill JF, et al. Effect of diet treatment on enuresis in children with migraine or hyperkinetic behavior. Clin Pediatr (Phila) 1992 May; 31(5):302-7; PMID: 1582098. *Not eligible target population*

61. Egger J, Carter CM, Soothill JF, et al. Oligoantigenic diet treatment of children with epilepsy and migraine. The Journal of pediatrics; 1989: 51-8. *Not eligible target population*

62. Egger J, Carter CM, Wilson J, et al. Is migraine food allergy? A double-blind controlled trial of oligoantigenic diet treatment. Lancet 1983 Oct 15; 2(8355):865-9; PMID: 6137694. *Not eligible exposure*

63. Egger J, McEwen L. Controlled study on the effectivity of hyposensitisation in children with food-induced migraine. Monatsschrift fur Kinderheilkunde; 1997: S21. *Language*

64. Egger J, Stolla A, McEwen L. Controlled study on the effectivity of hyposensibilisation due to enzyme potency in children with food-induced migraine. Monatsschrift fur Kinderheilkunde; 1992: 707. *Language*

65. Elkind AH, Wade A, Ishkanian G. Pharmacokinetics of frovatriptan in adolescent migraineurs. Journal of Clinical Pharmacology 2004 Oct; 44(10):1158-65; PMID: 15342617. *Not eligible outcomes*

66. Elser Jm WRC. Migraine headache in the infant and young child. Headache; 1990: 366-8. *Not eligible exposure*

67. Esposito SB, Gherpelli JL. Chronic daily headaches in children and adolescents: a study of clinical characteristics. Cephalalgia : an international journal of headache; 2004: 476-82. *Not eligible exposure*

68. Evers S, Rahmann A, Kraemer C, et al. Treatment of childhood migraine attacks with oral zolmitriptan and ibuprofen. Neurology 2006 Aug 8; 67(3):497-9; PMID: 16775229. *Not eligible target population*

69. Fernandez-Rodriguez CM, Lledo JL, Lopez-Serrano P, et al. [Effect of pentoxiphylline on survival, cardiac function, and portal and systemic hemodynamics in advanced alcoholic cirrhosis]. Revista Espanola de Enfermedades Digestivas; 2008: 481-9. *Language*

70. Forsythe WI, Redmond A. Two controlled trials of tyramine in children with migraine. Developmedchild Neurol; 1974: 794-9. *Not eligible exposure*

71. Fox AW. Clinical trial ethics. Headache 2005 Sep; 45(8):1090-1; author reply 1; PMID: 16109130. *Letter*

72. Freitag FG, Forde G, Neto W, et al. Analysis of pooled data from two pivotal controlled trials on the efficacy of topiramate in the prevention of migraine. J Am Osteopath Assoc 2007 Jul; 107(7):251-8; PMID: 17682112. *Not eligible target population*

73. Fujita M, Fujiwara J, Maki T, et al. The efficacy of sodium valproate and a MRA finding in confusional migraine. Brain & Development 2007 Apr; 29(3):178-81; PMID: 16973324. *Not eligible outcomes*

74. Gaby AR. Intravenous nutrient therapy: the "Myers' cocktail". Alternative Medicine Review 2002 Oct; 7(5):389-403; PMID: 12410623. *Not eligible target population*

75. Garaizar C, Prats JM, Zuazo E. [Results of prophylactic treatment for common childhood headaches]. Revista de Neurología; 1998. *Language*

76. Garaizar C, Prats JM, Zuazo E. [Response to prophylactic treatment of benign headache in children]. Revista de neurologia; 1998: 380-5. *Language*

77. Gillies D, Sills M, Forsythe I. Pizotifen (Sanomigran) in childhood migraine. A double-blind controlled trial. European neurology; 1986: 32-5. *Not eligible exposure*

78. Gobel H, Heinze A, Dworschak M, et al. Analgesic efficacy and tolerability of locally applied oleum menthae piperitae preparation LI 170 in patients with migraine or tension-type headache. Zeitschrift fur Allgemeinmedizin; 2001: 287-95. *Not eligible target population*

79. Gobel H, Heinze A, Dworschak M, et al. [Oleum menthae piperitae in the acute therapy of migraine and tension-type headache]. Zeitschrift fur Phytotherapie; 2004: 129-39. *Language*

80. Good PA, Taylor RH, Mortimer MJ. The use of tinted glasses in childhood migraine. Headache 1991 Sep; 31(8):533-6; PMID: 1960058. *Not eligible exposure*

81. Gottschling S, Meyer S, Gribova I, et al. Laser acupuncture in children with headache: a double-blind, randomized, bicenter, placebo-controlled trial. Pain; 2008: 405-12. *Not eligible exposure*

82. Gottschling S, Meyer S, Gribova I, et al. Laser acupuncture in children with headache: a double-blind, randomized, bicenter, placebo-controlled trial. Deutsche Zeitschrift fur Akupunktur; 2009: 52. *Not eligible exposure*

83. Greenlee CR, Puri V. Pediatric migraines: a case report. Journal of the Kentucky Medical Association 2003 Nov; 101(11):498-504; PMID: 14635578. *Not eligible outcomes*

84. Gruppo LQ, Jr. Intravenous Zofran for headache. Journal of Emergency Medicine 2006 Aug; 31(2):228-9; PMID: 17044590. *Not eligible target population*

85. Guariso G, Bertoli S, Cernetti R, et al. [Migraine and food intolerance: a controlled study in pediatric patients]. La Pediatria medica e chirurgica : Medical and surgical pediatrics; 1993: 57-61. *Language*

86. Gupta VK. Magnesium therapy for migraine: do we need more trials or more reflection? Headache 2004 May; 44(5):445-6; PMID: 15147256. *Comment*

87. Gysin T. [Clinical hypnotherapy/self-hypnosis for unspecified, chronic and episodic headache without migraine and other defined headaches in children and adolescents]. Forschende Komplementärmedizin; 1999: 44-6. *Language*

88. Gysin TZC. Clinical hypnosis therapy/self hypnosis for aspecific and episodic headache or migraine and other defined types of headaches in children and adolescents. Schweizerische Medizinische Wochenschrift Supplementum; 1994: 64-6. *Not eligible exposure*

89. Haddock CK, Rowan AB, Andrasik F, et al. Home-based behavioral treatments for chronic benign headache: a meta-analysis of controlled trials. Cephalalgia 1997 Apr; 17(2):113-8; PMID: 9137849. *Not eligible exposure*

90. Hall GC, Brown MM, Mo J, et al. Triptans in migraine: the risks of stroke, cardiovascular disease, and death in practice. Neurology 2004 Feb 24; 62(4):563-8; PMID: 14981171. *Not eligible exposure*

91. Hamalainen M, Jones M, Loftus J, et al. Sumatriptan nasal spray for migraine: a review of studies in patients aged 17 years and younger. International Journal of Clinical Practice 2002 Nov; 56(9):704-9; PMID: 12469987. *Not eligible exposure*

92. Hamalainen ML, Hoppu K, Santavuori P. Sumatriptan for migraine attacks in children: a randomized placebo-controlled study. Do children with migraine respond to oral sumatriptan differently from adults? Neurology 1997 Apr; 48(4):1100-3; PMID: 9109909. *Not eligible target population*

93. Hamalainen ML, Hoppu K, Santavuori PR. Oral dihydroergotamine for therapy-resistant migraine attacks in children. Pediatr Neurol 1997 Feb; 16(2):114-7; PMID: 9090684. *Not eligible target population*

94. Hershey AD. Adolescents with migraine: nature vs nurture. Neurology 2007 Jul 3; 69(1):12-3; PMID: 17606876. *Comment*

95. Hershey AD, Powers SW, Bentti AL, et al. Effectiveness of amitriptyline in the prophylactic management of childhood headaches. Headache 2000 Jul-Aug; 40(7):539-49; PMID: 10940092. *Not eligible outcomes*

96. Hershey AD, Powers SW, LeCates S, et al. Effectiveness of nasal sumatriptan in 5- to 12-year-old children. Headache 2001 Jul-Aug; 41(7):693-7; PMID: 11554957. *Not eligible target population*

97. Hershey AD, Powers SW, Vockell A-LB, et al. Coenzyme Q10 deficiency and response to supplementation in pediatric and adolescent migraine. Headache 2007 Jan; 47(1):73-80; PMID: 17355497. *Not eligible exposure*

98. Hirfanoglu T, Serdaroglu A, Gulbahar O, et al. Prophylactic drugs and cytokine and leptin levels in children with migraine. Pediatric Neurology 2009 Oct; 41(4):281-7; PMID: 19748048. *Not eligible outcomes*

99. Hoffman L, Mayzell G, Pedan A, et al. Evaluation of a monthly coverage maximum (drug-specific quantity limit) on the 5-HT1 agonists (triptans) and dihydroergotamine nasal spray. Journal of Managed Care Pharmacy 2003 Jul-Aug; 9(4):335-45; PMID: 14613452. *Not eligible exposure*

100. Holtmann M, Opp J, Tokarzewski M, et al. Human epilepsy, episodic ataxia type 2, and migraine. Lancet 2002 Jan 12; 359(9301):170-1; PMID: 11809294. *Comment*

101. Iannetti P, Spalice A, Iannetti L, et al. Residual and persistent Adie's pupil after pediatric ophthalmoplegic migraine. Pediatric Neurology 2009 Sep; 41(3):204-6; PMID: 19664538. *Not eligible outcomes*

102. Itil TM, Herrmann WM, Akpinar S. Prediction of psychotropic properties of lisuride hydrogen maleate by quantitative pharmaco-electroencephalogram. Int J Clin Pharmacol Biopharm 1975 Jul; 12(1-2):221-33; PMID: 1100539. *Not eligible target population*

103. Jeavons PM, Clark JE, Maheshwari MC. Treatment of generalized epilepsies of childhood and adolescence with sodium valproate ("epilim"). Dev Med Child Neurol 1977 Feb; 19(1):9-25; PMID: 403104. *Not eligible target population*

104. Kabbouche MA, Powers SW, Segers A, et al. Inpatient treatment of status migraine with dihydroergotamine in children and adolescents. Headache 2009 Jan; 49(1):106-9; PMID: 19125879. *Not eligible target population*

105. Kabbouche MA, Powers SW, Vockell A-LB, et al. Carnitine palmityltransferase II (CPT2) deficiency and migraine headache: two case reports. Headache 2003 May; 43(5):490-5; PMID: 12752755. *Not eligible target population*

106. Kabbouche MA, Vockell AL, LeCates SL, et al. Tolerability and effectiveness of prochlorperazine for intractable migraine in children. Pediatrics 2001 Apr; 107(4):E62; PMID: 11335783. *Not eligible target population*

107. Kakisaka Y, Wakusawa K, Haginoya K, et al. Abdominal migraine associated with ecchymosis of the legs and buttocks: does the symptom imply an unknown mechanism of migraine? Tohoku Journal of Experimental Medicine 2010; 221(1):49-51; PMID: 20453457. *Not eligible exposure*

108. Kitley JL, Lachmann HJ, Pinto A, et al. Neurologic manifestations of the cryopyrin-associated periodic syndrome. Neurology; 2010: 1267-70. *Not eligible target population*

109. Kmie, T., Kami, et al. [Usefulness of cerebral SPECT in the children with migraine]. Neurologia i neurochirurgia polska; 2005: S36-41. *Language*

110. Kornblau DH. Treatment of childhood migraine attacks with oral zolmitriptan and ibuprofen. Neurology 2007 Apr 24; 68(17):1441; PMID: 17452599. *Comment*

111. Korostenskaja M, Pardos M, Kujala T, et al. Impaired auditory information processing during acute migraine: a magnetoencephalography study. Int J Neurosci 2011 Jul; 121(7):355-65; PMID: 21425948. *Not eligible target population*

112. Kothare SV. Efficacy of flunarizine in the prophylaxis of cyclical vomiting syndrome and abdominal migraine. European Journal of Paediatric Neurology 2005; 9(1):23-6; PMID: 15701563. *Not eligible exposure*

113. Kroener-Herwig B, Denecke H. Cognitive-behavioral therapy of pediatric headache: are there differences in efficacy between a therapist-administered group training and a self-help format? J Psychosom Res 2002 Dec; 53(6):1107-14; PMID: 12479993. *Not eligible exposure*

114. Kung TA, Totonchi A, Eshraghi Y, et al. Review of pediatric migraine headaches refractory to medical management. Journal of Craniofacial Surgery 2009 Jan; 20(1):125-8; PMID: 19165008. *Not eligible outcomes*

115. Labbe E WDA. Temperature biofeedback in the treatment of children with migraine headaches. J Pediatr Psychol; 1983: 317-26. *Not eligible exposure*

116. Labbe EE. Treatment of childhood migraine with autogenic training and skin temperature biofeedback: a component analysis. Headache 1995 Jan; 35(1):10-3; PMID: 7868327. *Not eligible exposure*

117. Labbe EL, Williamson DA. Treatment of childhood migraine using autogenic feedback training. J Consult Clin Psychol 1984 Dec; 52(6):968-76; PMID: 6520289. *Not eligible exposure*

118. Lanzi G, D'Arrigo S, Termine C, et al. The effectiveness of hospitalization in the treatment of paediatric idiopathic headache patients. Psychopathology; 2007: 1-7. *Not eligible target population*

119. Larsson B, Carlsson J, Fichtel A, et al. Relaxation treatment of adolescent headache sufferers: results from a school-based replication series. Headache 2005 Jun; 45(6):692-704; PMID: 15953302. *Not eligible exposure*

120. Lastra L, Herranz J, Arteaga R. [Flunarizine or dihydroergotamine in the treatment of migraine in childhood. A randomised study of 50 patients.]. Anales Espa±oles de Pediatrfa.; 1990: 213-18. *Language*

121. Lastra Martinez L, Herranz Fernandez J, Arteaga Manjon Cabez R. [Flunarizine and dihydroergotamine in the treatment of migraine in children (published erratum appears in An Esp Pediatr 1990 Jun;32(6):566)]. An-Esp-Pediatr; 1990: 213-8. *Language*

122. Lastra Martínez L, Herranz Fernández J, Arteaga Manjón-Cabez R. [Flunarizine and dihydroergotamine in the treatment of migraine in children]. Anales españoles de pediatría; 1990: 213-8. *Language*

123. Lawler SP, Cameron LD. A randomized, controlled trial of massage therapy as a treatment for migraine. Ann Behav Med 2006 Aug; 32(1):50-9; PMID: 16827629. *Not eligible exposure*

124. Lehrer JF. Cyproheptadine's antiserotonin effects are responsible for its antimigraine activity. Headache 2004 Oct; 44(9):935; PMID: 15447711. *Comment*

125. Lewis D, Ashwal S, Hershey A, et al. Practice parameter: pharmacological treatment of migraine headache in children and adolescents: report of the American Academy of Neurology Quality Standards Subcommittee and the Practice Committee of the Child Neurology Society. Neurology 2004 Dec 28; 63(12):2215-24; PMID: 15623677. *Guideline*

126. Lewis DW. Please don't let her suffer like I did! Expert Review of Neurotherapeutics 2005 May; 5(3):291-4; PMID: 15938660. *Editorial*

127. Lewis DW. Headaches in children and adolescents. Pediatric Annals 2010 Jul; 39(7):388-90; PMID: 20666342. *Comment*

128. Lewis DW, Winner P, Hershey AD, et al. Efficacy of zolmitriptan nasal spray in adolescent migraine. Pediatrics 2007 Aug; 120(2):390-6; PMID: 17671066. *Not eligible target population*

129. Limmroth V, Biondi D, Pfeil J, et al. Topiramate in patients with episodic migraine: reducing the risk for chronic forms of headache. Headache 2007 Jan; 47(1):13-21; PMID: 17355489. *Not eligible target population*

130. Linder SL, Dowson AJ. Zolmitriptan provides effective migraine relief in adolescents. International Journal of Clinical Practice 2000 Sep; 54(7):466-9; PMID: 11070573. *Not eligible target population*

131. Linder SL, Mathew NT, Cady RK, et al. Efficacy and tolerability of almotriptan in adolescents: a randomized, double-blind, placebo-controlled trial. Headache 2008 Oct; 48(9):1326-36; PMID: 18484981. *Not eligible target population*

132. Lindkvist J, Airaksinen M, Kaukonen AM, et al. Evolution of paediatric off-label use after new significant medicines become available for adults: a study on triptans in Finnish children 1994-2007. Br J Clin Pharmacol 2011 Jun; 71(6):929-35; PMID: 21564161. *Not eligible target population*

133. Loder E. Safety of sumatriptan in pregnancy: a review of the data so far. CNS Drugs 2003; 17(1):1-7; PMID: 12467489. *Not eligible exposure*

134. Loder E, Goldstein R, Biondi D. Placebo effects in oral triptan trials: the scientific and ethical rationale for continued use of placebo controls. Cephalalgia 2005 Feb; 25(2):124-31; PMID: 15658949. *Not eligible target population*

135. Longo G, Rudoi I, Iannuccelli M, et al. [Treatment of essential headache in developmental age with L-5-HTP (cross over double-blind study versus placebo)]. La Pediatria medica e chirurgica : Medical and surgical pediatrics; 1984: 241-5. *Language*

136. Louis P, Schoenen J, Hedman C. Metoprolol v. clonidine in the prophylactic treatment of migraine. Cephalalgia 1985 Sep; 5(3):159-65; PMID: 3899370. *Not eligible target population*

137. Ludvigsson J. Letter: Propranolol in treatment of migraine in children. Lancet 1973 Oct 6; 2(7832):799; PMID: 4126507. *Letter*

138. Lutschg J, Vassella F. Flunarizine and propranolol in the treatment of migraine in children. Schweizerische Medizinische Wochenschrift; 1990: 1731-6. *Language*

139. Lütschg J, Vassella F. [The treatment of juvenile migraine using flunarizine or propranolol]. Schweizerische medizinische Wochenschrift; 1990: 1731-6. *Language*

140. MacLennan SC, Wade FM, Forrest KM, et al. High-dose riboflavin for migraine prophylaxis in children: a double-blind, randomized, placebo-controlled trial. J Child Neurol 2008 Nov; 23(11):1300-4; PMID: 18984840. *Not eligible exposure*

141. Maneyapanda SB, Venkatasubramanian A. Relationship between significant perinatal events and migraine severity. Pediatrics 2005 Oct; 116(4):e555-8; PMID: 16199683. *Not eligible exposure*

142. Martinez LL, Fernandez JH, Manjon-Cabeza RA. Flunarizine or dihydroergotamine in the treatment of migraine in childhood. A randomised study of 50 patients. <ORIGINAL> FLUNARIZINA O DIHIDROERGOTAMINA EN EL TRATAMIENTO DE LA MIGRANA EN LA INFANCIA. ESTUDIO RANDOMIZADO DE 50 PACIENTES. An Esp Pediat; 1990: 213-8. *Language*

143. Martinez-Lage JM. Flunarizine (Sibelium) in the prophylaxis of migraine. An open, long-term, multicenter trial. Cephalalgia 1988; 8 Suppl 8:15-20; PMID: 3052850. *Not eligible target population*

144. Mauskop A, Farkkila M, Hering-Hanit R, et al. Zolmitriptan is effective for the treatment of persistent and recurrent migraine headache. Curr Med Res Opin 1999; 15(4):282-9; PMID: 10640260. *Not eligible target population*

145. Mavromichalis I, Zaramboukas T, Giala MM. Migraine of gastrointestinal origin. European journal of pediatrics; 1995: 406-10. *Not eligible exposure*

146. Mazzone L, Vitiello B, Incorpora G, et al. Behavioural and temperamental characteristics of children and adolescents suffering from primary headache. Cephalalgia : an international journal of headache; 2006: 194-201. *Not eligible exposure*

147. McCarty J, Ruoff GE, Jacobson KD. Loracarbef (LY163892) versus cefaclor in the treatment of bacterial skin and skin-structure infections in an adult population. The American journal of medicine; 1992: 80s-5s. *Not eligible target population*

148. McGrath PJ, Humphreys P, Goodman JT, et al. Relaxation prophylaxis for childhood migraine: a randomized placebo-controlled trial. Dev Med Child Neurol 1988 Oct; 30(5):626-31; PMID: 3229560. *Not eligible exposure*

149. McGrath PJ, Humphreys P, Keene D, et al. The efficacy and efficiency of a self-administered treatment for adolescent migraine. Pain 1992 Jun; 49(3):321-4; PMID: 1408297. *Not eligible target population*

150. Mendizabal JE. Extended-release divalproex sodium improves the quality of life of adolescent migraineurs. Headache 2002 Apr; 42(4):327-8; PMID: 12010402. *Letter*

151. Miano S, Parisi P, Pelliccia A, et al. Melatonin to prevent migraine or tension-type headache in children. Neurol Sci 2008 Sep; 29(4):285-7; PMID: 18810607. *Not eligible exposure*

152. Mierzwi, ski J, Pawlak O, et al. [The vestibular system and migraine in children]. Otolaryngologia polska. The Polish otolaryngology; 2000: 537-40. *Language*

153. Moorjani BI, Rothner AD. Indomethacin-responsive headaches in children and adolescents. Seminars in Pediatric Neurology 2001 Mar; 8(1):40-5; PMID: 11332865. *Not eligible target population*

154. Moreno MJ, Abounader R, x00E, et al. Efficacy of the non-peptide CGRP receptor antagonist BIBN4096BS in blocking CGRP-induced dilations in human and bovine cerebral arteries: potential implications in acute migraine treatment. Neuropharmacology 2002 Mar; 42(4):568-76; PMID: 11955527. *Animal studies*

155. Morrato EH, Nicol GE, Maahs D, et al. Metabolic screening in children receiving antipsychotic drug treatment. Arch Pediatr Adolesc Med 2010 Apr; 164(4):344-51; PMID: 20368487. *Not eligible target population*

156. Natarajan S, Jabbour JT, Webster CJ, et al. Long-term tolerability of sumatriptan nasal spray in adolescent patients with migraine. Headache 2004 Nov-Dec; 44(10):969-77; PMID: 15546259. *Not eligible exposure*

157. Nezvalov, x00E, Henriksen K, et al. Triptan exposure during pregnancy and the risk of major congenital malformations and adverse pregnancy outcomes: results from the Norwegian Mother and Child Cohort Study. Headache 2010 Apr; 50(4):563-75; PMID: 20132339. *Not eligible target population*

158. Nickel AK, Hillecke T, Argstatter H, et al. Outcome research in music therapy: a step on the long road to an evidence-based treatment. Ann N Y Acad Sci 2005 Dec; 1060:283-93; PMID: 16597777. *Not eligible exposure*

159. Nicolodi M, Sicuteri F. L-5-hydroxytryptophan can prevent nociceptive disorders in man. Adv Exp Med Biol 1999; 467:177-82; PMID: 10721054. *Not eligible target population*

160. Noronha MJ. Double-blind randomised cross-over trial of timolol in migraine prophylaxis in children. Cephalalgia; 1985: 174-5. *Not eligible exposure*

161. Novembre E, Dini L, Bernardini R, et al. [Unusual reactions to food additives]. La Pediatria medica e chirurgica : Medical and surgical pediatrics; 1992: 39-42. *Language*

162. Oedegaard KJ, Riise T, Dilsaver SC, et al. A pharmaco-epidemiological study of migraine and antidepressant medications: complete one year data from the Norwegian population. J Affect Disord 2011 Mar; 129(1-3):198-204; PMID: 20889212. *Not eligible exposure*

163. Oelkers-Ax R, Leins A, Parzer P, et al. Butterbur root extract and music therapy in the prevention of childhood migraine: an explorative study. Eur J Pain 2008 Apr; 12(3):301-13; PMID: 17659990. *Not eligible exposure*

164. Ogose T, Manabe T, Abe T. Childhood steroid-responsive painful ophthalmoplegia: clues to ophthalmoplegic migraine. Journal of Pediatrics 2007 Aug; 151(2):e8-9; author reply e; PMID: 17643751. *Comment*

165. Olness K, Hall H, Rozniecki JJ, et al. Mast cell activation in children with migraine before and after training in self-regulation. Headache 1999 Feb; 39(2):101-7; PMID: 15613202. *Not eligible exposure*

166. Olness K, Hall H, Schmidt W, et al. Mast cell activation in child migraine patients before and after training in self regulation. Alternative therapies in health and medicine; 1997: 100-1. *Not eligible exposure*

167. Olness K, MacDonald J. Self-hypnosis and biofeedback in the management of juvenile migraine. J Dev Behav Pediatr 1981 Dec; 2(4):168-70; PMID: 7033294. *Not eligible exposure*

168. Olson AD, Li BUK. The diagnostic evaluation of children with cyclic vomiting: a cost-effectiveness assessment. Journal of Pediatrics 2002 Nov; 141(5):724-8; PMID: 12410206. *Not eligible target population*

169. Omata T, Takanashi J, Wada T, et al. Genetic diagnosis and acetazolamide treatment of familial hemiplegic migraine. Brain & Development 2011 Apr; 33(4):332-4; PMID: 20542393. *Not eligible target population*

170. O'Quinn S, Ephross SA, Williams V, et al. Pregnancy and perinatal outcomes in migraineurs using sumatriptan: a prospective study. Arch Gynecol Obstet 1999 Nov; 263(1-2):7-12; PMID: 10728620. *Not eligible exposure*

171. Osterhaus SO, Passchier J, van der Helm-Hylkema H, et al. Effects of behavioral psychophysiological treatment on schoolchildren with migraine in a nonclinical setting: predictors and process variables. J Pediatr Psychol 1993 Dec; 18(6):697-715; PMID: 8138865. *Not eligible exposure*

172. Ottman R, Lipton RB. Is the comorbidity of epilepsy and migraine due to a shared genetic susceptibility? Neurology 1996 Oct; 47(4):918-24; PMID: 8857719. *Not eligible exposure*

173. Overbeek WA, de Vroede MA, Lahuis BE, et al. [Antipsychotics and metabolic abnormalities in children and adolescents: a review of the literature and some recommendations]. Tijdschr Psychiatr 2010; 52(5):311-20; PMID: 20458678. *Language*

174. Paisley RD, Arora HS, Nazeri A, et al. Migraine and vasodepressor syncope in a large family. Texas Heart Institute Journal 2009; 36(5):468-9; PMID: 19876431. *Not eligible outcomes*

175. Pakalnis A, Kring D. Zonisamide prophylaxis in refractory pediatric headache. Headache 2006 May; 46(5):804-7; PMID: 16643584. *Not eligible outcomes*

176. Pakalnis A, Kring D, Paolicchi J. Parental satisfaction with sumatriptan nasal spray in childhood migraine. Journal of Child Neurology 2003 Nov; 18(11):772-5; PMID: 14696905. *Not eligible target population*

177. Panconesi A, Pavone E, Vacca F, et al. Triptans in the Italian population: a drug utilization study and a literature review. Journal of Headache & Pain 2008 Apr; 9(2):71-6; PMID: 18317865. *Not eligible exposure*

178. Parisi P, Kasteleijn-Nolst T, x00E, et al. A case with atypical childhood occipital epilepsy "Gastaut type": an ictal migraine manifestation with a good response to intravenous diazepam. Epilepsia 2007 Nov; 48(11):2181-6; PMID: 17711460. *Not eligible target population*

179. Parisi P, Pagani J, Galiffa S, et al. Migrainous vertigo unresponsive to antimigraine therapy in a child with "asymptomatic" cerebellar lesion: casual or causal association? Cephalalgia 2005 Oct; 25(10):831-5; PMID: 16162262. *Not eligible target population*

180. Parker GB, Pryor DS, Tupling H. Why does migraine improve during a clinical trial? Further results from a trial of cervical manipulation for migraine. Aust N Z J Med 1980 Apr; 10(2):192-8; PMID: 6992760. *Not eligible exposure*

181. Parker GB, Tupling H, Pryor DS. A controlled trial of cervical manipulation of migraine. Aust N Z J Med 1978 Dec; 8(6):589-93; PMID: 373735. *Not eligible target population*

182. Patrick DL, Hurst BC, Hughes J. Further development and testing of the migraine-specific quality of life (MSQOL) measure. Headache 2000 Jul-Aug; 40(7):550-60; PMID: 10940093. *Not eligible target population*

183. Pedersen E, Moller CE. Methysergide in migraine prophylaxis. Clinical pharmacology and therapeutics; 1966: 520-6. *Not eligible target population*

184. Pellock JM, Willmore LJ. A rational guide to routine blood monitoring in patients receiving antiepileptic drugs. Neurology 1991 Jul; 41(7):961-4; PMID: 2067658. *Editorial*

185. Philipp M. [Therapy of migraine. Clinical experience with Migraeflux, a new migraine drug]. Fortschritte der Medizin; 1977: 107-10. *Language*

186. Pintov S, Lahat E, Alstein M, et al. Acupuncture and the opioid system: implications in management of migraine. Pediatr Neurol 1997 Sep; 17(2):129-33; PMID: 9367292. *Not eligible exposure*

187. Piovesan EJ, Young Blood MR, Kowacs PA, et al. Prevalence of migraine in Noonan syndrome. Cephalalgia 2007 Apr; 27(4):330-5; PMID: 17376109. *Not eligible exposure*

188. Poston S, Dickson M, Johnsrud M, et al. Topiramate prescribing patterns among medicaid patients: diagnosis, comorbidities, and dosing. Clinical Therapeutics 2007 Mar; 29(3):504-18; PMID: 17577471. *Not eligible target population*

189. Pothmann R. Calcium-antagonist flunarizine vs. low-dose acetylsalicylic acid in childhood migraine: a double-blind study. Cephalalgia; 1985: 385-56. *Not eligible exposure*

190. Pothmann R. Migraine prophylaxis in children with low dose aspirin and flunarzin. Journal of Neurology; 1985: 219. *Record not found*

191. Pothmann R. Childhood migraine prophylaxis with calcium antagonist flunarizine and acetylsalicylic acid. A double blind study. Monatsschrift fur Kinderheilkunde; 1987: 646-9. *Language*

192. Pothmann R. [Prevention of migraine with flunarizine and acetylsalicylic acid. A double-blind study]. Monatsschrift Kinderheilkunde : Organ der Deutschen Gesellschaft für Kinderheilkunde; 1987: 646-9. *Language*

193. Pothmann R, Danesch U. Migraine prevention in children and adolescents: results of an open study with a special butterbur root extract. Headache 2005 Mar; 45(3):196-203; PMID: 15836592. *Not eligible exposure*

194. Pothmann R, Lobisch M. Acute treatment of episodic childhood tension-type headache with flupirtine and paracetamol - A double-blind crossover-study. Schmerz; 2000: 1-4. *Not eligible target population*

195. Pothmann R, Winter K. Migraine prophylaxis with dihydroergotamine - A double-blind placebo-controlled study. Cephalalgia Vol 9; 1989: 428-9. *Not eligible outcomes*

196. Pradalier A, Serratrice G, Collard M, et al. [Beta-blockers and migraine. Efficacy of time-release propranolol versus placebo]. Thérapie; 1990: 441-5. *Language*

197. Pradalier A, Serratrice G, Collard M, et al. Long-acting propranolol in migraine prophylaxis: results of a double-blind, placebo-controlled study. Cephalalgia 1989 Dec; 9(4):247-53; PMID: 2692838. *Not eligible target population*

198. Pradalier A, Vincent D. [Migraine and non-steroidal anti-inflammatory agents]. Pathologie-biologie; 1992: 397-405. *Language*

199. Rapoport A, Mauskop A, Diener HC, et al. Long-term migraine prevention with topiramate: open-label extension of pivotal trials. Headache 2006 Jul-Aug; 46(7):1151-60; PMID: 16866719. *Not eligible target population*

200. Riadh H, Mohamed G, Salah Y, et al. Pediatric case of ophthalmoplegic migraine with recurrent oculomotor nerve palsy. Canadian Journal of Ophthalmology 2010 Dec; 45(6):643; PMID: 21135898. *Not eligible exposure*

201. Richardson MS, Bowers BW, Petrie JL. The comparative clinical and economic benefits of drugs should be established and discussed as part of any formulary decision process. American Journal of Managed Care 2002 Aug; 8(8):693-4; author reply 4-5; PMID: 12212757. *Comment*

202. Richer LP, Laycock K, Millar K, et al. Treatment of children with migraine in emergency departments: national practice variation study. Pediatrics 2010 Jul; 126(1):e150-5; PMID: 20530076. *Not eligible target population*

203. Richter IL, McGrath PJ, Humphreys PJ, et al. Cognitive and relaxation treatment of paediatric migraine. Pain; 1986: 195-203. *Not eligible exposure*

204. Roach ES. Questioning botulinum toxin for headache: reality or illusion. Archives of Neurology 2008 Jan; 65(1):151-2; PMID: 18195157. *Comment*

205. Rompel H, Bauermeister PW. Aetiology of migraine and prevention with carbamazepine (Tegretol): results of a double-blind, cross-over study. S Afr Med J 1970 Jan 24; 44(4):75-80; PMID: 4905910. *Not eligible target population*

206. Rosen JA. Observations on the efficacy of propranolol for the prophylaxis of migraine. Ann Neurol 1983 Jan; 13(1):92-3; PMID: 6338806. *Not eligible target population*

207. Rosenberg MD, Strassels SA. Serotonin-active drugs. Journal of the Massachusetts Dental Society 2000; 48(4):48-50; PMID: 11819931. *Not eligible exposure*

208. Rothner AD, Wasiewski W, Winner P, et al. Zolmitriptan oral tablet in migraine treatment: high placebo responses in adolescents. Headache 2006 Jan; 46(1):101-9; PMID: 16412157. *Not eligible target population*

209. Rothner AD, Winner P, Nett R, et al. One-year tolerability and efficacy of sumatriptan nasal spray in adolescents with migraine: results of a multicenter, open-label study. Clinical Therapeutics 2000 Dec; 22(12):1533-46; PMID: 11192144. *Not eligible target population*

210. Ruiz C, Gener B, Garaizar C, et al. Episodic spontaneous hypothermia: a periodic childhood syndrome. Pediatric Neurology 2003 Apr; 28(4):304-6; PMID: 12849886. *Not eligible target population*

211. Salfield SA, Wardley BL, Houlsby WT, et al. Controlled study of exclusion of dietary vasoactive amines in migraine. Arch Dis Child 1987 May; 62(5):458-60; PMID: 3038036. *Not eligible exposure*

212. Salmon M. Pizotifen (BC.105. Sanomigran) in the prophylaxis of childhood migraine. Cephalalgia 1985; 5(Suppl 3):178; PMID. *Not eligible exposure*

213. Sánchez-Pérez R, Asensio M, Melchor A, et al. [Clinical features of migraine according to the questionnaire 'Alcoi-92' in the Comtat area]. Revista de neurologia; 1999: 459-63. *Language*

214. Santucci M, Cortelli P, Rossi PG, et al. L-5-hydroxytryptophan versus placebo in childhood migraine prophylaxis: a double-blind crossover study. Cephalalgia : an international journal of headache; 1986: 155-7. *Not eligible exposure*

215. Saper JR, Lake AE, Tepper SJ. Nefazodone for chronic daily headache prophylaxis: an open-label study. Headache 2001 May; 41(5):465-74; PMID: 11380644. *Not eligible exposure*

216. Sartory G, Muller B, Metsch J, et al. [Psychological and medicinal treatment of migraine in children and adolescents]. Verhaltenstherapie; 1995: A25. *Language*

217. Schabert E, Crow WT. Impact of osteopathic manipulative treatment on cost of care for patients with migraine headache: a retrospective review of patient records. Journal of the American Osteopathic Association 2009 Aug; 109(8):403-7; PMID: 19706829. *Not eligible exposure*

218. Scharff L, Marcus DA, Masek BJ. A controlled study of minimal-contact thermal biofeedback treatment in children with migraine. J Pediatr Psychol 2002 Mar; 27(2):109-19; PMID: 11821495. *Not eligible exposure*

219. Schradi A BJ. Results in the therapy of bronchial asthma using histaglobine. Zeitschrift fur Erkrankungen der Atmungsorgane, Mit Folia Bronchologica; 1972: 337-45. *Not eligible target population*

220. Seidel WT, Mitchell WG. Cognitive and behavioral effects of carbamazepine in children: data from benign rolandic epilepsy. Journal of child neurology; 1999: 716-23. *Not eligible target population*

221. Serdaroglu G, Erhan E, Tekgul H, et al. Sodium valproate prophylaxis in childhood migraine. Headache 2002 Sep; 42(8):819-22; PMID: 12390647. *Not eligible outcomes*

222. Sewell RA, Gottschalk CH. Problem child is no headache. Headache 2011 Feb; 51(2):306; author reply -7; PMID: 21083559. *Comment*

223. Shin JI, Lee JS. Can chronic fatigue symptoms associated with nutcracker phenomenon be treated with aspirin? Medical Hypotheses 2007; 69(3):704-5; PMID: 17329037. *Comment*

224. Shuhaiber S, Pastuszak A, Schick B, et al. Pregnancy outcome following first trimester exposure to sumatriptan. Neurology 1998 Aug; 51(2):581-3; PMID: 9710039. *Not eligible exposure*

225. Shulman ST. Headaches! Pediatric Annals 2010 Jul; 39(7):386-7; PMID: 20666341. *Comment*

226. Sicuteri F, Del Bene E. The influence of tryptophan and parachlorophenylalanine on the sexual activity in man. Acta vitaminologica et enzymologica; 1975: 100-2. *Not eligible target population*

227. Silberstein SD, Loder E, Forde G, et al. The impact of migraine on daily activities: effect of topiramate compared with placebo. Curr Med Res Opin 2006 Jun; 22(6):1021-9; PMID: 16846536. *Not eligible target population*

228. Silberstein SD, Neto W, Schmitt J, et al. Topiramate in migraine prevention: results of a large controlled trial. Arch Neurol 2004 Apr; 61(4):490-5; PMID: 15096395. *Not eligible target population*

229. Silcocks P, Whitham D, Whitehouse WP. P3MC: a double blind parallel group randomised placebo controlled trial of Propranolol and Pizotifen in preventing migraine in children. Trials 2010; 11:71; PMID: 20553601. *Not eligible exposure*

230. Sillanpää M, Koponen M. Papaverine in the prophylaxis of migraine and other vascular headache in children. Acta paediatrica Scandinavica; 1978: 209-12. *Not eligible exposure*

231. Siniatchkin M, Hierundar A, Kropp P, et al. Self-regulation of slow cortical potentials in children with migraine: an exploratory study. Applied Psychophysiology and Biofeedback; 2000: 13-32. *Not eligible target population*

232. Sorge F, De Simone R, Marano E, et al. Efficacy of flunarizine in the prophylaxis if migraine in children: a double-blind, cross-over, controlled study. Cephalalgia; 1985: 174. *Not eligible exposure*

233. Soriani S, Battistella PA, Naccarella C, et al. Nimesulide and acetaminophen for the treatment of juvenile migraine: A study for comparison of efficacy, safety, and tolerability. Headache Quarterly; 2001: 233-6. *Not eligible target population*

234. Spigt MG, Kuijper EC, Schayck CP, et al. Increasing the daily water intake for the prophylactic treatment of headache: a pilot trial. European journal of neurology : the official journal of the European Federation of Neurological Societies; 2005: 715-8. *Not eligible exposure*

235. Sri-udomkajorn S, Ruangsuwan S. Short-term outcomes of tension type and migraine headache in children. Journal of the Medical Association of Thailand 2008 Oct; 91 Suppl 3:S104-8; PMID: 19253504. *Not eligible outcomes*

236. Storey JR, Calder CS, Hart DE, et al. Topiramate in migraine prevention: a double-blind, placebo-controlled study. Headache 2001 Nov-Dec; 41(10):968-75; PMID: 11903524. *Not eligible target population*

237. Swanson JW. Topiramate for migraine prevention. Curr Neurol Neurosci Rep 2005 Mar; 5(2):77-8; PMID: 15743542. *Not eligible target population*

238. Symon DN, Russell G. Double blind placebo controlled trial of pizotifen syrup in the treatment of abdominal migraine. Arch Dis Child 1995 Jan; 72(1):48-50; PMID: 7717738. *Not eligible exposure*

239. Teixeira AL, Meira FC, Maia DP, et al. Migraine headache in patients with Sydenham's chorea. Cephalalgia : an international journal of headache; 2005: 542-4. *Not eligible target population*

240. Tepper SJ, Donnan GA, Dowson AJ, et al. A long-term study to maximise migraine relief with zolmitriptan. Curr Med Res Opin 1999; 15(4):254-71; PMID: 10640258. *Not eligible target population*

241. Terwindt GM, Ophoff RA, Haan J, et al. Familial hemiplegic migraine: a clinical comparison of families linked and unlinked to chromosome 19.DMG RG. Cephalalgia : an international journal of headache; 1996: 153-5. *Not eligible target population*

242. Titus F, Davalos A, Alom J, et al. 5-Hydroxytryptophan versus methysergide in the prophylaxis of migraine. Randomized clinical trial. Eur Neurol 1986; 25(5):327-9; PMID: 3536521. *Not eligible exposure*

243. Torelli P, Cologno D, Manzoni GC. Weekend headache: a retrospective study in migraine without aura and episodic tension-type headache. Headache 1999 Jan; 39(1):11-20; PMID: 15613189. *Not eligible exposure*

244. Trottier ED, Bailey B, Dauphin-Pierre S, et al. Practice variation after implementation of a protocol for migraines in children. European Journal of Emergency Medicine 2010 Oct; 17(5):290-2; PMID: 19864956. *Not eligible target population*

245. Trottier ED, Bailey B, Dauphin-Pierre S, et al. Clinical outcomes of children treated with intravenous prochlorperazine for migraine in a pediatric emergency department. J Emerg Med 2010 Aug; 39(2):166-73; PMID: 19150192. *Not eligible target population*

246. Tuchin PJ, Pollard H, Bonello R. A randomized controlled trial of chiropractic spinal manipulative therapy for migraine. J Manipulative Physiol Ther 2000 Feb; 23(2):91-5; PMID: 10714533. *Not eligible target population*

247. Tuchman M, Edvinsson L, Geraud G, et al. Zolmitriptan provides consistent migraine relief when used in the long-term. Curr Med Res Opin 1999; 15(4):272-81; PMID: 10640259. *Not eligible target population*

248. Ueberall M. Sumatriptan in paediatric and adolescent migraine. Cephalalgia 2001; 21 Suppl 1:21-4; PMID: 11678817. *Not eligible exposure*

249. Uldall P, Bulteau C, Pedersen S, et al. Single-blind study of safety, tolerability, and preliminary efficacy of tiagabine as adjunctive treatment of children with epilepsy. Epilepsia 1995; 36(Suppl 3):S147-S8; PMID. *Not eligible target population*

250. Vardi Y, Rabey IM, Streifler M, et al. Migraine attacks. Alleviation by an inhibitor of prostaglandin synthesis and action. Neurology; 1976: 447-50. *Not eligible target population*

251. Vasconcellos E, Pina-Garza JE, Millan EJ, et al. Analgesic rebound headache in children and adolescents. J Child Neurol 1998 Sep; 13(9):443-7; PMID: 9733291. *Not eligible target population*

252. Verspeelt J, De Locht P, Amery WK. Post-marketing cohort study comparing the safety and efficacy of flunarizine and propranolol in the prophylaxis of migraine. Cephalalgia 1996 Aug; 16(5):328-36; discussion 288; PMID: 8869768. *Not eligible exposure*

253. Victor S, Ryan SW. Drugs for preventing migraine headaches in children. Cochrane Database of Systematic Reviews 2003; (4):CD002761; PMID: 14583952. *Not eligible outcomes*

254. Vieira J, x00E, Pedro, et al. Ophthalmoplegic migraine and infundibular dilatation of a cerebral artery. Headache 2008 Oct; 48(9):1372-4; PMID: 18631189. *Not eligible exposure*

255. Virtanen R, Aromaa M, Rautava P, et al. Changing headache from preschool age to puberty. A controlled study. Cephalalgia : an international journal of headache; 2007: 294-303. *Not eligible outcomes*

256. Visudtibhan A, Lusawat A, Chiemchanya S, et al. Flunarizine for prophylactic treatment of childhood migraine. Journal of the Medical Association of Thailand 2004 Dec; 87(12):1466-70; PMID: 15822542. *Not eligible exposure*

257. Visudtibhan A, Thampratankul L, Khongkhatithum C, et al. Migraine in junior high-school students: A prospective 3-academic-year cohort study. Brain & Development 2010 Nov; 32(10):855-62; PMID: 20060252. *Not eligible outcomes*

258. Vollono C, Ferraro D, Miliucci R, et al. The abnormal recovery cycle of somatosensory evoked potential components in children with migraine can be reversed by topiramate. Cephalalgia 2010 Jan; 30(1):17-26; PMID: 19489886. *Not eligible target population*

259. Vonderheid-Guth B, Todorova A, Wedekind W, et al. Evidence for neuronal dysfunction in migraine: concurrence between specific qEEG findings and clinical drug response--a retrospective analysis. European Journal of Medical Research 2000 Nov 30; 5(11):473-83; PMID: 11121368. *Not eligible exposure*

260. Wainscott G, Sullivan FM, Volans GN, et al. The outcome of pregnancy in women suffering from migraine. Postgrad Med J 1978 Feb; 54(628):98-102; PMID: 634879. *Not eligible exposure*

261. Wang S-J, Fuh J-L, Lu S-R, et al. Outcomes and predictors of chronic daily headache in adolescents: a 2-year longitudinal study. Neurology 2007 Feb 20; 68(8):591-6; PMID: 17182975. *Not eligible outcomes*

262. Weaver MB, Mackowiak JI, Solari PG. Triptan therapy impacts health and productivity. Journal of Occupational & Environmental Medicine 2004 Aug; 46(8):812-7; PMID: 15300133. *Not eligible target population*

263. Wilkins AJ, Patel R, Adjamian P, et al. Tinted spectacles and visually sensitive migraine. Cephalalgia 2002 Nov; 22(9):711-9; PMID: 12421156. *Not eligible exposure*

264. Winner P, Dalessio D, Mathew N, et al. Concomitant administration of antiemetics is not necessary with intramuscular dihydroergotamine. The American journal of emergency medicine; 1994: 138-41. *Not eligible target population*

265. Wober C, Wober-Bingol C. Intranasal sumatriptan for the acute treatment of migraine in children. Neurology 2000 Mar 14; 54(5):1209-10; PMID: 10720311. *Not eligible target population*

266. Young WB, Hopkins MM, Shechter AL, et al. Topiramate: a case series study in migraine prophylaxis. Cephalalgia 2002 Oct; 22(8):659-63; PMID: 12383061. *Not eligible target population*

267. Zafeiriou DI, Vargiami E. Childhood steroid-responsive painful opthalmoplegia: clues to opthalmoplegic migraine. Journal of Pediatrics 2006 Dec; 149(6):881; PMID: 17137913. *Not eligible target population*

268. Zangaladze A, Asadi-Pooya AA, Ashkenazi A, et al. Sporadic hemiplegic migraine and epilepsy associated with CACNA1A gene mutation. Epilepsy & Behavior 2010 Feb; 17(2):293-5; PMID: 20071244. *Not eligible target population*

269. Zgorzalewicz M. [Visual evoked potentials in children and school adolescents with migraine and tension-type headache. Clinical and neurophysiological correlations]. Neurologia i neurochirurgia polska; 2005: S26-35. *Language*

270. Zwozdziak W. [Treatment of migraine with migristin]. Wiadomości lekarskie (Warsaw, Poland : 1960); 1973: 1617-20. *Language*